TESTIMONIALS

"Recently I asked Medium Paul to use one of his Vogel Wands to clear a psychic attack that was affecting my lungs and my mobility. I could barely walk. Even though I am in Canada and he is in Brazil, he was able to energetically remove the attack without seeing me in person."
—Gene, Toronto, Ontario Province, Canada

"There was a tornado supercell that came out of Arkansas and into Kentucky. Watching the live Doppler radar on TV, I could see the storm was getting close, about 30 minutes from my house. Immediately I started to do the Severe Weather Mitigation that Medium Paul recommends. Watching on TV, I could see the tornado start to dissipate in real time. Within 15 minutes the storm was completely weakened. The weatherman said he couldn't believe it."
—Heather, Louisville, Kentucky

"My sister Griselda was having severe respiratory problems and was in the ICU. The doctors advised us to prepare for the worse. Medium Paul did distance energy work and telepathically appealed to Griselda's motherly instincts by connecting Griselda to her five-year-old son. The next morning Griselda came out of the coma. It is now nine years later, and she remains healthy and fine."
—Monica, Buenos Aires, Argentina

"I have known Medium Paul for over 10 years. He ha guided me through a serious, life-threatening illness. His innate intuition is very high and accurate. But combined with the use of his invocations, he has taught me how to move out of seriously negative and destructive energy territory and completely clear them from working against me and my healing. He knows how to personalize and resolve any situation large or small with use of his energy practices and highly specific invocations. My healing has been maximized in each instance through working with him."   —Dana, Tucson, Arizona

"In 2016 I had lung cancer and an aortic aneurism. A CT scan showed a high level of arterial plaque. My surgeon was very concerned about the risk of a stroke or heart attack. For two months before my scheduled surgery, I worked with Medium Paul. Besides helping me spiritually, he focused on the arterial plaque. When my surgeon opened my heart, he was surprised to find an absence of arterial plaque. It's eight years later and I'm still alive and well."

—Gaudêncio, Brasilia, Brazil

"I am a psychic reader and life coach. I was about to have my third thyroid surgery. The gland had grown as big as a grapefruit and was endangering my airway. If I had surgery, there was a chance I would lose my voice completely. Doctors said it was risky but had to be done. I spoke to Medium Paul. He said he would clear the negative energy in the operating room, my body, the surgeon, the hospital, and any and all other aspects of the case. After five hours of surgery, I emerged and was immediately able to speak. I am still improving day by day. I am sure Medium Paul's work made a strong and positive difference in the outcome."

—Deborah, Charleston, West Virginia

"Recently Medium Paul did some energy work on me remotely (from over 4,000 miles away). I am 28 now. For 16 years I have been plagued with anorexia and bulimia. I have been to therapists, in-patient and out-patient programs, taken dozens of different medications. Nothing has worked. About a week after Medium Paul did energy work me, my bulimia was completely gone. More time has passed, and I have not experienced any of the old urges and cravings. My life has truly changed." — Rose, Phoenix, Arizona

"After half a century of pain and standing crooked I now am able to stand erect without any pain at all."

—Hans, Los Angeles, California

"Each and every time I have reached out to Medium Paul, he has done energy work, a clearing, and a relationship reset. I am not certain how it works, but it does. The guidance he has given me has helped me make decisions that I might not otherwise have made. Paul's specificity and wisdom are profound."

—Nora, Albany, New York

"My granddaughter, Micaela, was seriously ill and unable to breathe on her own. At the hospital she was intubated and administered oxygen directly into her lungs. The doctors said she had a serious case of pneumonia and was getting worse by the minute. He advised us to pray! At that point I knew that I needed some real help. I contacted my sister in Brazil and Medium Paul began energy treatments immediately. The next day I went to the hospital. As the elevator doors opened a doctor emerged with a great smile on his face! Michaela was breathing on her own again. She would make a full recovery soon. I know that Paul is not a common man. I feel that he is a saint or a light worker of some kind because he works miracles. I can never thank him enough!"

—Elva, Buenos Aires, Argentina

"A few days ago Medium Paul asked for my assistance in conducting an experiment for him to remotely improve the qualities and taste of Trader Joe's "Two Buck Chuck", Charles Shaw wine, to reflect the aroma and taste of far superior wines. Medium Paul called from Brazil to my home in the Napa Valley. Two bottles each of Charles Shaw Chardonnay and Cabernet had been purchased at Trader Joe's the previous day. A bottle of Chardonnay and one of Cabernet was placed to my left as "control" samples. The remaining two bottles were placed on my right, identified as the "Subject" wines. Medium Paul then went through an oral process to remove impurities, defects in taste and quality, and to enhance the subject wines to reflect the aroma and profile of superior wines. I have a degree in Viticulture and Oenology, extensive experience managing wineries, and have lived in wine country the majority of my life. By the time Medium Paul was finished, I was speechless to confirm that he had transformed completely the subject wines, resulting in unique and pleasurable flavor profiles. I have never seen such a thing since."

—Jeffrey, Napa, California

MORE BOOKS FROM
THE SAGER GROUP

*Shaman: The Mysterious Life and Impeccable
Death of Carlos Castaneda*
by Mike Sager

*Sarabeth and the Five Spirits: A Novel about Channeling,
Consciousness, Healing and Murder*
by Beth Gineris

Meeting Mozart: A Novel Drawn from the Secret Diaries of Lorenzo Da Ponte
by Howard Jay Smith

Death Came Swiftly: A Novel About the Tay Bridge Disaster of 1879
by Bill Abrams

*The Deadliest Man Alive: Count Dante, The Mob
and the War for American Martial Arts*
by Benji Feldheim

Lifeboat No. 8: Surviving the Titanic
by Elizabeth Kaye

*The Pope of Pot: And Other True Stories of Marijuana
and Related High Jinks*
by Mike Sager

See our entire library at TheSagerGroup.net

THE MASTER INVOCATIONS

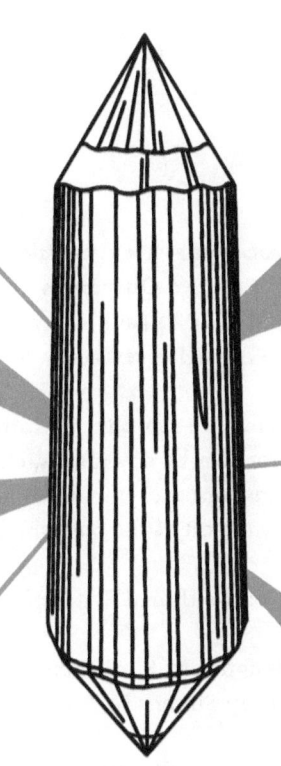

Moving Energy to Achieve
Positive Outcomes

PAUL HARRY SIMONS

**The Master Invocations: Moving Energy to Achieve
Positive Outcomes**
Copyright © 2024 Paul Harry Simons
All rights reserved.

Published in the United States of America.

Cover and Interior Designed by Siori Kitajima, PatternBased.com
Photo of Paul Harry Simons by Paula Rocha Nogueira

Cataloging-in-Publication data for this book is available from the Library of
Congress
ISBN-13s
eBook: 978-1-958861-27-1
Paperback: 978-1-958861-28-8
Hardcover: 978-1-958861-29-5

Published by The Sager Group LLC
(TheSagerGroup.net)

THE MASTER INVOCATIONS

Moving Energy to Achieve
Positive Outcomes

PAUL HARRY SIMONS

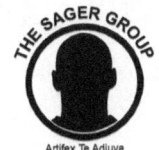

THE SAGER GROUP

Artifex Te Adiuva

CONTENTS

FOREWORD

It is important to be aware that the invocations and the information provided in this book is 100% "in the Light" and cannot be used for negative purposes. There are spiritual safeguards built in; any and all attempts to use the information in this book to harm anything or anyone will bounce back to the sender before it can set up or take effect.

There is absolutely no dogma associated with this healing modality, you will never be asked to adopt a belief system. Your religious views, race, nationality, sexual orientation, political affiliation, and core values are never questioned or even discussed.

AUTHOR'S NOTE

In 2019 I was hospitalized for infection in both kidneys and treated intravenously. During the hospitalization, I started blacking out for one to two seconds at a time—something that had never happened to me before. An exam was promptly scheduled, and it showed I had an aneurysm in my aorta. My prognosis was grim. I had a 93% chance of mortality and only a 7% chance of survival.

A CT scan of the chest brought more bad news. My aortic valve was failing. In addition to fixing the aneurysm, doctor needed to perform a valve transplant. The procedures were scheduled for the coming week.

I knew this operation was going to be extremely complex, so I used a Vogel Wand to perform a variety of invocations to prepare for surgery and to aid the surgeons. The following are the invocations I performed before the surgeries and as needed while hospitalized:

Attachments
Cloaking
Grounding
Hospital
Patient Room
Pre-Op Surgery
Psychic Surgery
Faith
Blood Transfusion

Some of these invocations were done daily. Others were performed less frequently.

To begin, I performed three different invocations on myself, in order to clear my own personal energy. The Attachment invocation removed any extraneous negative entities and attachments. Subsequently, I invoked the Cloaking in order to energetically shield me from any spirits in other realms that might be seeking to harm me. The third was the Grounding invocation, which centered my energy within my own body. After these three invocations were completed, I was at my best and able to focus on further clearings at the medical facility.

In general, I knew that hospitals energetically contain a lot of residual pain and suffering left over from previous patients and their various medical issues. I also knew the facility needed to be cleared of that trauma, so I used the Hospital invocation to clear the entire medical facility.

Next, I used the Patient Room invocation for my room. The invocation included all medical equipment and furnishings. Can you imagine the traumatic energy left behind after a previous patient experienced a painful death, now embedded in the same mattress and bed that I was occupying? Even wiping the bed and mattress down with alcohol and disinfecting it still would not clear the traumatic energy. Everything in the room had to be cleared: the bed, mattress, IV stands, side tables, chairs, food trays, and bathroom fixtures.

After my room was cleared it felt lighter and had a more comfortable feel. The cleaning staff, food service workers and some nurses commented that they felt a presence in my room that they didn't feel anywhere else on the hospital ward.

Next I used the Pre-Op Surgery invocation to energetically clear the operating room. Imagine the traumatic energy left behind in an operating table that has been used daily for 25 years, multiple times a day. The same for the instruments and devices, IV stands, and other medical equipment. All of these things have also absorbed trauma repeatedly and have probably never been cleared energetically.

Then I used the Psychic Surgery invocation to assist the surgeon. I need to make this very clear: the *surgeon* did the surgery. I did not have anything to do with the physical surgery. What the invocation did, however, was to channel all of the spiritual energy of the Ascended Masters and Angelic Beings *through* the surgeon. Ascended Masters and Angelic Beings don't make mistakes — so when they were teamed up with the surgeon's skills, we were then able to achieve the best possible outcome.

The Faith invocation helped to raise my positivity to the highest levels when the outcome was pending and during ongoing care. I will give an example: During the course of my recovery, I had to have my sternum amputated due to a bacterial infection. I was put on two different intravenous antibiotics for 45 days. I was in excruciating pain, having been cut from the Adam's apple to the belly button and having had all of the connected ribs severed at the sternum. However, since I was in faith, and not fear, I was able to reduce the need for a strong prescription opiate and instead use an over-the-counter pain medication.

The Blood Transfusion invocation helped me to first clear the donor's soul connection from the blood. Then I matched the energetic vibration of the transfusion to my own blood's unique frequency. You can be sure that the blood you receive from a transfusion has a vibration, but it is very likely not to be anything close to your own blood's frequency. Upon the introduction of the donor's soul into your body, you don't want that soul fighting with yours for control of *your* body.

In each of my surgeries there was a high risk of complications — up to and including death. Yet I was able to undergo and survive four open heart surgeries in the short span of one month.

Now, several years later I have beaten a 7% survival rate, and I am healthy, fully functional and living a normal life.

I do not think I would be alive today if I had not performed these invocations with the Vogel Wand. This is the reason I have decided to share The Master Invocations with the public.

Feel free to contact me at MediumPaul.com if you have any questions.

—Paul Harry Simons

ACKNOWLEDGEMENTS

I am immeasurably grateful to Marcel Vogel. His lifetime achievements are many, including his pioneering work at IBM. In his retirement, he developed the Vogel Wand healing modality. Marcel's love, dedication and energy was put into documenting, training and teaching the first generation of Vogel Wand light workers. He paved the way for humanity's ascension at the cusp of the Age of Aquarius.

I thank my cardiac surgeons, Dr. Cláudio Ribeiro da Cunha, Dr. Jéssica Silva Silvério, and Dr. Elson Borges Lima who performed a total of four open-heart surgeries on me in February and March of 2019.

I also would like to give special thanks to some key spiritual friends: Astrologer Jane Sezak, of Kapaa, HI, who introduced me to astrology in August 1978. In addition, I thank Dr. Lester Adler; Brad, Michael and David; Fred Rusher; Anita Dalton; and Lauralea Adkins, all of Sedona, AZ; Medium and trans-channel Kevin Ryerson of San Francisco, CA; Ray Queiroga Pinto of Belo Horizonte, Minas Gerais, Brazil, the master lapidary craftsman who custom makes all of my Vogel Wands.

Finally, I recognize Ribomar Cavalcante, of Anapolis, Goias, Brazil for always answering my questions about spiritual, cultural, regional and provincial matters in Brazil; Valerie Laconto of Scottsdale, AZ for her friendship, kindness and assistance during the writing of this book; Gene Meyer, for the help and assistance he provided; my maternal grandfather, the late Harry Jacob Eisenberg, who told me at an early age "The harder you work, the luckier you get"; and most importantly, my wife, Perla Simons, who has always been here for me and has had unwavering faith, both in the good times and the difficult moments. For all of this, I am blessed and eternally grateful.

DISCLAIMER

The reader understands that all information contained within this book is subject to personal interpretation. The author shall not be held liable for any interpretations or decisions made by recipients based on information provided. All invocations and written material included in this book are spiritually based and not intended to replace qualified medical, legal, or financial advice.

INTRODUCTION

What are Master Invocations?

Invocations are powerful methods to move and clear energy for creating the best possible outcomes. In some instances, fear, trauma, and anxiety, which are embedded in a person, can be released, so that life improves. People may be in these emotions because they are not grounded. They have trouble manifesting and accomplishing their goals. The grounding invocation merges the soul of the person with the physical body. Once that invocation is complete, that person can reach their maximum potential.

There are 72 invocations broken down into 12 chapters covering many different subjects. Select the appropriate invocation for what is needed to accomplish. Sometimes there is more than one invocation needed to accomplish your objective.

Note: It takes a lot of experience to know which invocations to use on yourself or others. The more you work, the better you get at identifying the correct invocation in each situation. You will not be an expert from reading this book, but you will gain a good foundation. You won't be a master Vogel Crystal Wand healer just by reading this book. It takes years of practice to fully understand how to approach the different situations you will have.

What do they do?

The invocations in this book employ the use of thought and speech to move energy. They have highly specific language and recitation techniques for directing, cleansing, balancing, eradicating, or increasing energy in any given situation.

Moving Energy

The invocations change outcomes for the better by moving energy. There are many ways to move energy. For example, talking and thinking are ways most people move energy daily. Everybody does this and anyone can do the invocations in this book. In this modality, we use two ways to move energy; extracting it and projecting it.

Energy is moved in many ways. Reiki, for example, moves energy by the use of symbols that run universal life force frequencies through the practitioner's hands either in person or telepathically at a distance. Acupuncture moves energy through the body along meridian points. Energy also moves through speech and thinking.

What is the difference between Vogel crystal wand invocations, the Rosary (Roman Catholic), or prayers? Or any other type of energy work?

This modality uses a very specific set of instructions to invoke an outcome. These invocations are very focused and defined which makes it much clearer to the Ascended Masters and Angelic Beings what is desired and needs to be accomplished. As for other forms of manifestation such as prayer, or using the Rosary (Roman Catholic), the desired outcome can sometimes be generalized and vague.

How to use the Invocations

The invocations in this book depend on these three qualities:
1. Mediumship
2. Invocation and intention
3. The Vogel Crystal Wand or telepathic projection

To begin, the medium sets the intention, reads an invocation, and immediately begins moving energy and changing outcomes. Intention is the major factor in achieving results.

Sixty-five of the invocations in this book include both projecting and extracting energy. These seven invocations need only to project energy to accomplish the desired outcome: Cloaking, Grounding, Soul Code Activation, Earthbound Spirits, Bone Marrow, Charging Minerals, and Projecting Minerals.

The more evolved and experienced the medium is, the more advanced the work will be. The amount of spiritual past lives one has had, and the underlying soul consciousness will guide your work and results.

When you start reading the individual invocations, you will see two arrow icons. While using the Vogel Wand, you must wave the wand in the air before you in a circular motion, clockwise (for projecting) or counterclockwise (for extracting). The projecting arrow icon ⟳ represents the wand circling in a clockwise direction. The extracting arrow icon ⟲ represents an arrow circling in a counterclockwise direction. These two arrow logos are clearly marked both at the start and during each of the invocations, so you can achieve the results you are seeking. Telepathically, you can say the invocation and it automatically projects or extracts because your mind's eye understands whether it needs projecting or extracting.

Do you recite the invocations out loud?

The invocations can be spoken out loud or telepathically. Depending on the location and situation you may be able or unable to speak an invocation out loud. For example, at a funeral, you may clear the people gathered of pain and trauma telepathically to not interrupt the blessings being said by the person officiating at the funeral.

Do you have to use a wand?

The short answer is no, you can project the intention of the invocation telepathically without a Vogel Wand. However, you increase the cohesion many times over when you use a Vogel Wand because it focuses the energy.

Choosing the proper invocation

It is important to choose the appropriate invocation. This book is organized by chapters so it is easier to find the invocation by subject/category.

The completeness of the invocation you are using is critical too, so you must be thorough and not leave anything out of your invocation to get the best outcome. Finally, the Vogel Crystal Wand or telepathic projection along with your experience and working knowledge of how to perform the work is the driver.

Cohesion

The cohesion, which is the amount of power driving the invocation, can be increased if you use a highly focused Vogel Crystal Wand. This makes the invocation more powerful but isn't necessary to achieve the results you are seeking.

You may be curious: how and why does a Vogel Crystal Wand increase cohesion? The answer is that the Vogel Wand is a crystal cut to sacred geometry which amplifies the intention you are projecting or extracting.

Purchasing a wand — what you need to know

Where can you get a Vogel Crystal Wand? They are sold on many online platforms; however, buyer beware, it is widely believed that up to 95% of the crystals sold as "Vogel Crystal Wands" or "Vogel-Inspired Wands" are not cut to the precise sacred geometry needed to create the stronger cohesion. You *can* use a crystal cut incorrectly, however, it will *not* give you the extra cohesion, so it is important to acquire your Vogel Wand from a reputable source.

I would suggest purchasing from either a crystal dealer online or in a brick-and-mortar store that specializes in Vogel Wands and has gotten the Vogels from a Vogel Wand manufacturer which cut the wands to the sacred geometry angles specified by Marcel Vogel.

How to clean and care for your wand

To clean the Vogel of any energy charge it may have picked up while being used, you can use breath, the way Marcel Vogel cleared wands, a horseshoe magnet, or an electro-magnetic tape eraser. You can also clear the Vogel telepathically with intention.

Note: Do not use water to clear your Vogel wand because if the temperature is even one degree higher or lower than the Vogel wand it will cause it to contract or expand, possibly fracturing the Vogel.

Salt can also cause fracturing at the faceting, so never use salt to clear a Vogel. Also, crystal and Tibetan singing bowls and tuning forks can fracture a Vogel Wand, so do not use these sound healing modalities around your Vogel Wand.

The Vogel Crystal Wand is a neutral instrument that creates highly directed cohesion and should never hold an energy charge. Therefore, the Vogel should not be placed in sunlight or moonlight. This is the opposite of what is typically done with most crystals which hold a vibration and are charged up to project the inherent frequency and charge that specific mineral vibrates at. With Vogels, the invocation is the charge, and is the delivery methodology to move the energy.

When you buy your first Vogel wand, you will have many options to choose from. There will be several different lengths, number of facets, quartz with or without inclusions, various types of facet cuts, and earth-mined or laboratory quartz options. You don't need the most expensive, fanciest Vogel Wand. I believe using an inexpensive 3-4" long end-to-end Vogel with 12 or 24 facets is sufficient. At my training workshops, I offer 24-sided Vogels with inclusions for the participants because that provides enough cohesion and is reasonably priced.

Education and Training

As part of my life's work, I created this book to make the knowledge and information I have learned, channeled, and perfected over many decades available to the general public, especially light workers.

I teach introductory and advanced Vogel Crystal Wand Practitioner Workshops. I use this book as the workbook for these training programs. You can also contact me to schedule private consultations or training, in the English language. Information on current offerings is available on my website: www.MediumPaul.com.

STARTING THE ENERGY CLEARING WORK

Attachments

The first invocations are to clear attachments and cloaking the energy field. You will want to perform these clearings on yourself before working on anyone else. It is important to understand why we pick up and accumulate attachments, so let me explain.

Everyone interacts dynamically with other people. We project and receive cords, attachments, and hooks from the people we are interacting with. Over time this accumulates, and we are "wired and corded" to all the people and their attachments. This distorts our soul blueprint, in both positive and negative ways. It alters our true nature and the frequency we vibrate at, our mediumship abilities, and many other variables. Sometimes people say they are "under stress" or overwhelmed with their life and daily responsibilities. Often what is really going on is they have too many cords pulling them in multiple directions. When we clear attachments, we are removing all the connections to other people and spirits. After being cleared, you return to your essence, your true soul's nature.

When a person is cleared of cords, attachments, implants, hooks, entities, and thought forms, we are bringing the client back to their original nature. This is who they are, and in the vibration and frequency they are incarnated in and are supposed to be living in. This clearing immediately lifts tension and stress out of the person, and they usually feel lighter. The muscular-skeletal and nervous systems are also more aligned. Often, after a clearing, if you stretch or shrug your shoulders, you will notice that your muscles and bones are a lot looser and more relaxed and clearer of tension.

I equate clearing attachments with the daily function of bathing or taking a shower. We need to wash and clean our physical body regularly, and so it is with our energetic body.

Another aspect of attachment clearings that applies to some people is if they take strong prescription medication, pain killers, opiates, or drink a lot of alcoholic beverages, they accumulate attachments. This can affect a person's clarity of mind, decision-making process, and even, in extreme cases, can turn into a form of possession. The attachment clearing eliminates these attachments. However, if you clear a person of attachments who is a recreational drug user, heavy drinker, or who takes strong prescription medication, pain killers, or opiates and they reintroduce the drugs or alcohol, the attachments can return.

I use very specific invocations which involve a Vogel Crystal Wand for both projecting and clearing to remove attachments. If you are interested in my work and would like to book a session, please go to the scheduling page on my website, MediumPaul.com.

Cloaking

Cloaking is a method to make your energy signature invisible to both incarnate beings (people, animals) and discarnate spirits. When you cloak yourself and your aura, your overall energy is completely undetectable. There are two aspects to cloaking that, when combined, produce the result.

In the first, you make holographic duplicates of yourself that look like you, feel like you, and seem to be you, but have no connection to your soul. When you send out trillions and trillions of these holographic duplicates all over the universe. anybody or anything looking for you will connect to a holographic duplicate, essentially a decoy of you. Since the holographic duplicates are not connected to you, nothing actually makes its way back to you.

In the second aspect to cloaking, you obscure your own aura and energy signature by placing trillions and trillions of mirrored sacred geometry symbols all around you. With the mirrored sacred geometry, it's impossible to identify your aura or energy, with a few exceptions (we will discuss the exceptions at the end).

Cloaking doesn't work when you are physically connected—for instance shaking someone's hand or hugging them. Physical contact connects you with another person's energy, so avoid physical contact if you want your aura and energy to be fully undetected and don't want other people's energy to transfer into you.

Grounding

After clearing attachments and cloaking yourself or the other person, it is very important to be grounded in order to manifest and accomplish your goals. When our soul is "in our body," we are physically more coordinated and can focus clearly and execute very complex tasks. When a person is not grounded, they are more susceptible to misjudging or miscalculating decisions or daily activities, which can lead to accidents. When a person is grounded, they are very present, listen more intently, and have fewer misunderstandings or miscommunications.

Soul Code Activation

The soul code activation invocation can be used to raise a person's vibration and increase energy in all their cellular DNA. This invocation "lights up" a person's aura by downloading galactic light code through the physical body, thereby raising the consciousness to a higher frequency. The heart chakra opens more completely in higher dimensions, and this creates a softening of the dense energy a person may otherwise exhibit.

UNDERSTANDING DIFFERENT TYPES OF CLEARINGS

Antiques and Secondhand Jewelry

It is not commonly understood, nor generally known by the average person, that there are recorded memories stored in antiques, second-hand jewelry, and "hand-me-downs" (used items). If these items are not energetically cleared of the people who owned and used the item, the energy of the original owner(s) will come through.

For instance, In 2008 I was given an 1845 antique, fold down secretary desk with three wooden drawers. It was beautiful. I brought it into my house and immediately felt a strange serpent energy in the lower part of the desk. Upon meditating and tuning into this energy, I discovered the original owner was an Arizona farmer and this desk had been in his farmhouse.

One day the farmer heard his wife screaming and ran into the farmhouse. She told him she had been bitten by a snake hiding in the bottom drawer. The farmer grabbed a shovel and killed the snake.

The spirit of the snake was still earthbound and stayed connected with the desk, even 160 years later. I did an energy clearing of the desk and crossed the snake into the light. Afterward, the desk was in a collapsed, and zero-point neutral state, and I was comfortable using this wonderful antique for many years.

While antique jewelry is sentimental and often very beautiful, it needs to be cleared to avoid passing on problems or issues from the original owner(s). There is memory and energy stored in EVERY antique and secondhand jewelry item. Antiques carry with them memories of everything that happened to an item since it was made. Most likely the attached memory is neutral, but often there are events where traumatic emotional charges were imprinted in the antique or jewelry.

When second hand or family heirloom jewelry is passed down to descendants, the energy of the people who wore the jewelry is stored in the metal, stones, pearls, and settings.

Every person has distinct unique energy. For example, a diamond wedding ring that was worn for forty-five years would carry a lot of emotional and energetic charges. When a new owner of the ring wears it, they are receiving the energetic charge of everything that happened to the original owner of the ring. No matter how beautiful the piece is, I strongly recommend clearing the energy stored in the ring before another person wears it.

It is very easy to energetically clear antiques and secondhand jewelry using Vogel Crystal Wands. The clearing will permanently remove the emotional charges and bring the item to a collapsed and zero-point neutral state, so that it can bond with a new owner, completely clear of the old emotional charges. There is no reason to not have heirloom jewelry, "hand me downs," or antiques, as they often have significant sentimental meaning. Also, many antiques are no longer made or manufactured using the same techniques as in the past. Just be aware that each piece has a full memory of the history that has occurred around it. Be sure to energetically clear it with a Vogel Crystal Wand.

Earthbound Spirits

I have worked on helping earthbound spirits cross into the light. Accidents, sudden "unnatural" deaths, murders, and suicides can result in a spirit being stuck earthbound and unable to cross into the light by themselves.

The ego many times does not allow the spirit to transcend because of unfinished business, emotions, trauma. When a spirit is earthbound the ego is present as if they were still alive, so their mode of thinking is the same.

I have found it helpful to ask ancestors and pets who have crossed over to come back to assist the earthbound spirit to cross. Often the earthbound spirit is confused and basically lost. When they see family members whom they knew, as well as beloved long-dead pets come to them, they are happy to go with the family members or pets into the light. It is instantaneous and joyous when the family and pets come and assist the earthbound spirit to cross.

In accidental deaths, often the earthbound spirit feels responsible to stay for various reasons. Sometimes a parent who is an earthbound spirit wants to see their children grow up, sometimes it a spouse who is earthbound and wants to stay around to protect the spouse who is still incarnated. In these cases, the family members and pets are very, very helpful in making it easier to move on and go into the light.

In suicides, the shock of sudden death often results in deep regret, anguish, guilt, and strong emotions, holding the earthbound spirit and keeping it stuck. They can literally be earthbound indefinitely; it is always better for the earthbound spirit to cross so they prepare for their next incarnation.

With murder victims, there is often shock, anger, turmoil, and a desire to seek revenge or "justice" for what happened to them. In one case, I worked on a woman who was murdered and left on the side of an Interstate in 2005.

When I was brought into the case in 2017, I asked the earthbound spirit of the woman, "Why are you staying there, on the side of the interstate?"

"I'm waiting for the three men who murdered me to return," she said."

I then asked her "Do you know how long have you been waiting for them?"

"Not that long," she responded.

When I told her it had been twelve years since her murder, and that the three men were probably not coming back, she was utterly surprised. She had no idea it had been so long. Then I suggested it might be time for her to cross, and she did.

More often than not, I feel, earthbound spirits need help to cross. They are not here to cause problems for the living, as we often believe. Instead, they are here because they had a sudden or traumatic death and didn't get the help they needed to cross into the light.

We can help these earthbound spirits. There is no better tool for this than a Vogel Crystal Wand. Often this type of work is pro bono (free). While there is no financial compensation, we will know we helped a forgotten soul. To me that's compensation enough.

Homicide

Homicides are complex and can require multiple clearings.

There was a murder on a bus not far from my home in Brazil. The bus driver was stabbed multiple times and died in the driver's seat. As a result, there were three different Homicide clearings needed.

First, the bus needed clearing. Obviously, after such a violent incident there is a tremendous amount of trauma remaining in the bus itself. Because he bus company didn't have a spare bus to replace immediately replace this bus, I did a clearing. Afterward the bus continued to be used on the same route for two months, until a new bus was purchased and put into service to replace it.

After I cleared the bus, I did a second clearing on all the passengers who took the bus. All the frequent passengers who took this bus route knew a murder had occurred on this bus and these people had a lot of fear and anxiety about riding on it, so a clearing helped allay their fears.

Finally, I did a third clearing of the physical location where the bus had been when the murder took place, I cleared that space of the trauma and negative emotional charge that remained there.

Additionally, the homicide victim needs to be cleared and crossed into the light if they are earthbound. Please refer to the earthbound spirit invocation for the homicide victim.

Virus, Vaccines, and Boosters

There are some innovative approaches to Virus Mitigation Clearings of great interest, such as before virus symptoms from previously infected people who do not feel 100% recovered.

These virus mitigation energy clearings are distinctive and unique from all other work I am familiar with. I used the initial approach of channeling galactic energy through the individual and replaced the low vibrational virus frequency in their cellular DNA with a higher galactic light code. This gets the energy moving on a cellular level, but it's only part of what needs to be done to clear out the virus energetically. Much more needs to be addressed, especially the energetic paralysis from fear.

When low vibration energy is replaced with higher frequency, you need to consider several factors in whether the person can benefit from this holistic energy approach. There is processing time involved in almost every case, and sometimes the person receiving the energy infusion needs adaption time to "rewire energetically" to handle the higher vibrational energy. Also, in some cases, a person is too unstable, ungrounded, and cannot hold the higher frequency, so doesn't fully recover.

Each case needs to be looked at individually because everybody is different energetically. This is an essential basis to work from. However, there is free will, and every outcome is unique.

I use the Vogel Crystal Wand with very specific invocations for both projecting and clearing to remove attachments.

Recently we have had an unprecedented number of fatal virus cases. I found out that there appears to be about 25% to 30% residual virus in people who test negative; why? Low vibrational residual energy needs to be energetically cleared out and replaced with a higher vibrational light code. Residual virus energy is the low vibrational energy of the virus variant that is still stuck in the body, usually in specific organs. It can be almost paralyzing and slow down recovery because low vibrational energy is slow to heal and doesn't always fully heal. I found residual virus mitigation clearings need to be done when a person has pain in a specific organ or area of the body that isn't going away. I replace the stuck, low vibration residual energy by running a high vibrational galactic light code through the residual virus frequency. This clears the paralysis and allows rapid recovery and healing.

I find that being in faith really helps to speed up the healing process, knowing that you will make a full recovery, and holding these thoughts reduce the time needed to make your recovery. People sick with a virus who are in fear will slow down or stop the recovery process. So it's very, very important to reside in Faith, not in fear while you are going through the recovery process.

In addition to replacing the residual energy, I discovered another issue that often keeps the recovering person from making a full recovery. A percentage of the people aware that the sick person is in recovery project fear, anxiety, and trauma at the ill person. This comes from family, friends, coworkers, social media contacts, and others who know the person. People projecting onto the sick person create a form of energetic paralysis that prevents full recovery and can "lock-in" residual low vibrational energy; this needs to be cleared when identified.

What needs to be done is to immediately clear out all the cords and attachments from these family, friends, coworkers, social media contacts, and other people who know about the sick person's condition and then cloak the person so that this fear, anxiety, and trauma does not reattach.

Genetic Lineage and Ancestral DNA

Everybody's cellular DNA has genetic lineage memory stored and sometimes this helps elevate a person to accomplish more but other times there is a memory that makes it impossible to achieve success. Deep clearing of the genetic lineage helps to free a person up so they are not limited by memories that interfere with current goals and aspirations.

- Do you constantly have money problems?
- Is your love life not working out?
- Do you find yourself repeating the same patterns?
- Do you keep attracting "bad boys" or "gold diggers" you know aren't good for you?
- Are you struggling to keep up financially and can't figure out why things never work out?

These are all themes which could indicate coded ancestral DNA and coded lineage programming passed down from your bloodline creating outcomes you do not want.

There are emotional charges passed down from your ancestors through maternal and paternal lineage which create stress, tension, trauma, and anxiety. This emotional charge is a coded memory of events that happened to an earlier generation in your ancestry resulting in difficulty and trauma.

An example of this would be if your great-grandfather owned a bank in 1929 and it failed at the start of the Great Depression. The emotional charge in his body created by the trauma of financial failure could have been passed down to your grandparent, and further down to your own parent, eventually effecting your own body and state of being as coded emotional memory in your nervous system, DNA, and genetics.

This ancestral trauma affecting your immediate family could potentially cause your own insecurities and challenges with business endeavors, struggle with financial independence, and extreme difficulty getting or holding employment.

The good news is that this coded memory can be cleared out of your DNA! You do not have to be victim to this type of programming, memory, and trauma any longer. By clearing out the coded memory in your DNA/genetics, you can stop this cycle for good and prevent it from being passed down to future generations.

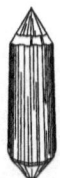

CHAPTER 1

UNIVERSAL CLEARINGS

ATTACHMENTS

◗ (Projecting) We are placing _____(Name) in an orb with mirrors facing in and mirrors facing out; the Sirius B Council on the outside and Archangels Raphael, Uriel, Gabriel, and Michael at the four cardinal points.

We are placing an orb to the right of the main orb with mirrors facing in and mirrors facing out, the Sirius B Council on the outside, Archangels Raphael, Uriel, Gabriel, and Michael at the four cardinal points.

We invoke all of the Ascended Masters and Angelic Beings of the Universe, to go up as a conduit, through the Galactic Core, Central Sun, Secret Sun, Platinum Sun, and come down into conscious, subconscious, and all altered states of consciousness into _____(Name).

◖ (Extracting) We are clearing _____(Name), of all attachments, from the manifest to the unmanifest, from particle to wave, transmuting to a neutral energy. Clearing all EMF-energy fluctuations from solar flares and geomagnetic storms, cellular transmissions, and all forms of radiation, in matter, dark matter, antimatter, energy, space, time, and all alternate realities, mind control, non-beneficial interdimensional beings, earthbound tricksters, extraterrestrials, artificial intelligence, subliminal messages, hypnosis and posthypnotic suggestions in all forms, parasites, viruses, non-beneficial bacteria, collective-consciousness fear, anxiety, trauma, emotional charges, cords, attachments, implants, hooks, entities, and thought forms, seen or unseen, cloaked or uncloaked, in conscious, subconscious, and all altered states of consciousness, even if they are changing frequencies and dimensions, simultaneously, in matter, dark matter, antimatter, energy, space, time, and all alternate realities. We are moving everything into the containment orb at the count of 10.

1, 2, 3, 4, 5, 6, 7, 8, 9, 10 - increasing the cohesion to the 987th Fibonacci number.

We are clearing all imprints, echoes, residuals, energetic tattoos associated with what we just cleared, simultaneously, in matter, dark matter, antimatter, energy, space, time, and all alternate realities. We are moving everything into the containment orb at the count of 10.

1, 2, 3, 4, 5, 6, 7, 8, 9, 10 - increasing the cohesion to the 987th Fibonacci number.

(Projecting) We are sealing the containment orb.

(Extracting) Sending it to the Central Sun.

And so it is, and so it is, and so it is.

CLOAKING

◯ (Projecting) We are creating 987 trillion holographic duplicates of _____(Name) all across the universe, simultaneously, in matter, dark matter, antimatter, energy, space, time, and all alternate realities.

The holographic duplicates are identical but not energetically connected to _____(Name) in any way.

We are creating 987 trillion holographic mirrored orbs, triangles, merkabas, pyramids, Christ chambers over, under, and around _____(Name) on a fractal, atomic, and cellular level, simultaneously, in matter, dark matter, antimatter, energy, space, time, and all alternate realities, cloaking and making _____(Name) holographically invisible in the spirit realms on a fractal, atomic, and cellular level, simultaneously, in matter, dark matter, antimatter, energy, space, time, and all alternate realities now.

And so it is, and so it is, and so it is.

FAITH

☋ (Projecting) We are placing _____(Name) in an orb with mirrors facing in and mirrors facing out; the Sirius B Council on the outside and Archangels Raphael, Uriel, Gabriel, and Michael at the four cardinal points.

We are placing a containment orb to the right of the main orb with mirrors facing in and mirrors facing out, the Sirius B Council on the outside, Archangels Raphael, Uriel, Gabriel, and Michael at the four cardinal points.

We invoke all of the Ascended Masters and Angelic Beings of the Universe, to go up as a conduit, through the Galactic Core, Central Sun, Secret Sun, Platinum Sun, and come down into conscious, subconscious, and all altered states of consciousness into _____(Name).

☋ (Extracting) We are clearing _____(Name) of all fear-based programming, removing fight-and-flight trauma stored in the cellular DNA from any traumas still held in the physical body in matter, dark matter, antimatter, energy, space, time, and all alternate realities, from the manifest to the unmanifest, from particle to wave, transmuting to a neutral energy. Clearing all EMF energy fluctuations from solar flares and geomagnetic storms, cellular transmissions, and all forms of radiation, in matter, dark matter, antimatter, energy, space, time, and all alternate realities, mind control, non-beneficial interdimensional beings, earthbound tricksters, extraterrestrials, artificial intelligence, subliminal messages, hypnosis, and posthypnotic suggestions in all forms, parasites, viruses, non-beneficial bacteria, collective-consciousness fear, anxiety, trauma, emotional charges, cords, attachments, implants, hooks, entities, and thought forms, seen or unseen, cloaked or uncloaked, in conscious, subconscious, and all altered states of consciousness, even if they are changing frequencies and dimensions, simultaneously, in matter,

dark matter, antimatter, energy, space, time, and all alternate realities. We are moving everything into the containment orb at the count of 10.

1, 2, 3, 4, 5, 6, 7, 8, 9, 10 - increasing the cohesion to the 987th Fibonacci number.

We are clearing all imprints, echoes, residuals, energetic tattoos associated with what we just cleared, simultaneously, in matter, dark matter, antimatter, energy, space, time, and all alternate realities. We are moving everything into the containment orb at the count of 10.

1, 2, 3, 4, 5, 6, 7, 8, 9, 10 - increasing the cohesion to the 987th Fibonacci number.

◗ (Projecting) We are sealing the containment orb.

◖ (Extracting) Sending it to the Central Sun.

◗ (Projecting) We invoke all the Ascended Masters and Angelic Beings of the Universe to go up as a conduit, through the Galactic Core, Central Sun, Secret Sun, Platinum Sun, into conscious, subconscious, and all altered states of consciousness, to work through _____(Name) eyes, ears, mind, and hands in Faith for the best possible outcome in all facets of this incarnation.

And so it is, and so it is, and so it is.

FILTERING SPIRITS

◔ (Projecting) We are placing an orb around _____(Name) with mirrors facing in and mirrors facing out, the Sirius B Council on the outside, Archangels Raphael, Uriel, Gabriel, and Michael at the four cardinal points.

We are placing a containment orb to the right of the main orb with mirrors facing in and mirrors facing out, the Sirius B Council on the outside, Archangels Raphael, Uriel, Gabriel, and Michael at the four cardinal points.

We invoke all the Ascended Masters and Angelic Beings of the Universe, to go up as a conduit, through the Galactic Core, Central Sun, Secret Sun, Platinum Sun, and come down into conscious, subconscious, and all altered states of consciousness into _____(Name).

◔ (Extracting) We are clearing _____(Name) from low-vibrational entities and demons, as well as fear, anxiety, and trauma, from the manifest to the unmanifest, from particle to wave, transmuting to a neutral energy. Clearing all EMF energy fluctuations from solar flares and geomagnetic storms, cellular transmissions, and all forms of radiation, in matter, dark matter, antimatter, energy, space, time, and all alternate realities, mind control, non-beneficial interdimensional beings, earthbound tricksters, extraterrestrials, artificial intelligence, subliminal messages, hypnosis, and posthypnotic suggestions in all forms, parasites, viruses, non-beneficial bacteria, collective-consciousness fear, anxiety, trauma, emotional charges, cords, attachments, implants, hooks, entities, and thought forms, seen or unseen, cloaked or uncloaked, in conscious, subconscious, and all altered states of consciousness even if they are changing frequencies and dimensions, simultaneously, in matter, dark matter, antimatter, energy, space, time, and all alternate realities. We are moving everything into the containment orb at the count of 10.

1, 2, 3, 4, 5, 6, 7, 8, 9, 10 – increasing the cohesion to the 987th Fibonacci number.

We are clearing all imprints, echoes, residuals, energetic tattoos associated with what we just cleared, simultaneously, in matter, dark matter, antimatter, energy, space, time, and all alternate realities. We are moving everything into the containment orb at the count of 10.

1, 2, 3, 4, 5, 6, 7, 8, 9, 10 – increasing the cohesion to the 987th Fibonacci number.

◐ (Projecting) We are sealing the containment orb.

◐ (Extracting) Sending it to the Central Sun.

◐ (Projecting) We invoke all the Ascended Masters and Angelic Beings of the Universe to go up as a conduit, through the Galactic Core, Central Sun, Secret Sun, Platinum Sun, into conscious, subconscious, and all altered states of consciousness, and raise the vibration of the immediate area around _____(Name) to the highest frequency at which it can vibrate and to keep all low-vibrational entities and demons away from _____(Name) on a perpetual basis.

And so it is, and so it is, and so it is.

GROUNDING

◑ (Projecting) We are placing gold, electric ultraviolet blue, platinum and plasma light codes in _____(Name) Heart Chakra, making a vertical toric field using the infinity symbol. Starting at the Heart Chakra, we go down to the present dimension of the center of the New Earth, the crystal core of the Mother, and back up through the Heart Chakra, continuing to the Galactic Core. Now we are making a second toric field, a 3-foot-wide horizontal column of gold, electric ultraviolet blue, platinum and plasma light code, center-lined on the Heart Chakra, and taking the 3-foot-wide column of light vertically down to the present dimension of the center of the New Earth, the crystal core of the Mother, then back up through the Heart Chakra to the Galactic Core, grounding and connecting _____(Name) to the unified field.

To reinforce the grounding, we invoke all of the Ascended Masters and Angelic Beings of the Universe, to go up as a conduit through the Galactic Core, Central Sun, Secret Sun, Platinum Sun, in conscious, subconscious, and all altered states of consciousness and taking Ruby Red light and eucalyptus saplings, go down through the Crown, Third Eye, Throat, Heart, Solar Plexus, Sacral, and Root Chakras to the present dimension of the center of the New Earth, the crystal core of the Mother.

And so it is, and so it is, and so it is.

SOUL CODE ACTIVATION

◯ (Projecting) We are placing _____(Name) in the center of a 6-sided star in a tunnel of light code, moving in a clockwise direction, morphing into a place I call a temple of light code, a large luminous place with light emanating from the floor, the walls and the ceiling. There is a 13-pointed gold star on the ceiling, a 13-pointed gold star on the floor. _____(Name) is seated in the center of the temple of light code with a big Selenite crystal holographically in front of (him/her/them), I am seated on the other side holographically as a facilitator. Glittering, shimmering light is connecting the points of the star above with the points of the star below as they continue to move in a clockwise direction, and now we are morphing into the center of a holographic gold star with 987 points, now we are going into the Galactic Core and activating _____(Name) soul codes.

And so it is, and so it is, and so it is.

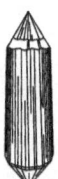

CHAPTER 2

PROPERTY AND LOCATIONS

ANTIQUES AND SECONDHAND JEWELRY

↻ (Projecting) We are placing an orb around the antiques and/ or secondhand jewelry with mirrors facing in and mirrors facing out, the Sirius B Council on the outside, Archangels Raphael, Uriel, Gabriel, and Michael at the four cardinal points.

We are placing a containment orb to the right of the main orb with mirrors facing in and mirrors facing out, the Sirius B Council on the outside, Archangels Raphael, Uriel, Gabriel, and Michael at the four cardinal points.

We invoke all the Ascended Masters and Angelic Beings of the Universe, to go up as a conduit through the Galactic Core, Central Sun, Secret Sun, Platinum Sun, into conscious, subconscious, and all altered states of consciousness, and come down into the antiques and/or secondhand jewelry.

☾ (Extracting) We are clearing _____(Name of Antique or Second Hand Jewelry), from the manifest to the unmanifest, from particle to wave, transmuting to a neutral energy. Clearing all EMF energy fluctuations from solar flares and geomagnetic storms, cellular transmissions, and all forms of radiation, in matter, dark matter, antimatter, energy, space, time and all alternate realities, mind control, non-beneficial interdimensional beings, earthbound trick-sters, extraterrestrials, artificial intelligence, subliminal messages, hypnosis and posthypnotic suggestions in all forms, parasites, viruses, non-beneficial bacteria, collective-consciousness fear, anxiety, trauma, emotional charges, cords, attachments, implants, hooks, entities, and thought forms, seen or unseen, cloaked or uncloaked, in conscious, subconscious, and all altered states of consciousness, even if they are changing frequencies and dimensions, simultaneously, in matter, dark matter, antimatter, energy, space, time, and all alternate

realities. We are moving everything into the containment orb at the count of 10.

1, 2, 3, 4, 5, 6, 7, 8, 9, 10 - Increasing the cohesion to the 987th Fibonacci number.

We are clearing all imprints, echoes, residuals, energetic tattoos associated with what we just cleared, simultaneously, in matter, dark matter, antimatter, energy, space, time, and all alternate realities. We are moving everything into the containment orb at the count of 10.

1, 2, 3, 4, 5, 6, 7, 8, 9, 10 - Increasing the cohesion to the 987th Fibonacci number.

◝ (Projecting) We are sealing the containment orb.

◜ (Extracting) Sending it to the Central Sun.

And so it is, and so it is, and so it is.

BAR AND LOUNGE

◗ (Projecting) We are placing _____(Name) in an orb with mirrors facing in and mirrors facing out, the Sirius B Council on the outside, Archangels Raphael, Uriel, Gabriel, and Michael at the four cardinal points.

We are placing a containment orb to the right of the main orb with mirrors facing in and mirrors facing out, the Sirius B Council on the outside, Archangels Raphael, Uriel, Gabriel, and Michael at the four cardinal points.

We invoke all the Ascended Masters and Angelic Beings of the Universe, to go up as a conduit, through the Galactic Core, Central Sun, Secret Sun, Platinum Sun, into conscious, subconscious, and all altered states of consciousness, and come down into _____ (Name).

◖ (Extracting) We are clearing the parking lot outside, the bar and lounge, furniture, fixtures, equipment, and all surfaces of the building, including inside, of interpersonal conflicts or negative energy between the people who work there, as well as all customers, from the manifest to the unmanifest, from particle to wave, transmuting to a neutral energy. Clearing all EMF energy fluctuations from solar flares and geomagnetic storms, cellular transmissions, and all forms of radiation, in matter, dark matter, antimatter, energy, space, time, and all alternate realities, mind control, non-beneficial interdimensional beings, earthbound tricksters, extraterrestrials, artificial intelligence, subliminal messages, hypnosis and posthypnotic suggestions in all forms, parasites, viruses, non-beneficial bacteria, collective-consciousness fear, anxiety, trauma, emotional charges, cords, attachments, alcohol, drug, and all other implants, hooks, entities, and thought forms, seen or unseen, cloaked or uncloaked, in conscious, subconscious, and all altered states of consciousness, even if they are changing frequencies and dimensions, simultaneously, in matter, dark matter, antimatter, energy, space, time, and all alternate realities. We are moving everything into the containment orb at the count of 10.

1, 2, 3, 4, 5, 6, 7, 8, 9, 10 - Increasing the cohesion to the 987th Fibonacci number.

We are clearing all imprints, echoes, residuals, energetic tattoos associated with what we just cleared, simultaneously, in matter, dark matter, antimatter, energy, space, time, and all alternate realities. We are moving everything into the containment orb at the count of 10.

1, 2, 3, 4, 5, 6, 7, 8, 9, 10 - Increasing the cohesion to the 987th Fibonacci number.

↷ (Projecting) We are sealing the containment orb.

↶ (Extracting) Sending it to the Central Sun.

And so it is, and so it is, and so it is.

COLLECTIVE CONSCIOUSNESS

☽ (Projecting) We are placing _____(Specific Collective Consciousness) in an orb with mirrors facing in and mirrors facing out, the Sirius B Council on the outside, Archangels Raphael, Uriel, Gabriel, and Michael at the four cardinal points.

We are placing a containment orb to the right of the main orb with mirrors facing in and mirrors facing out, the Sirius B Council on the outside, Archangels Raphael, Uriel, Gabriel, and Michael at the four cardinal points.

We invoke all the Ascended Masters and Angelic Beings of the Universe, to go up as a conduit through the Galactic Core, Central Sun, Secret Sun, Platinum Sun into conscious, subconscious, and all altered states of consciousness, and come down into _____ (Specific Collective Consciousness).

☾ (Extracting) We are clearing fear, anxiety, and trauma that _____(Specific Collective Consciousness) has internalized, from the manifest to the unmanifest, from particle to wave, transmuting to a neutral energy. Clearing all EMF energy fluctuations from solar flares and geomagnetic storms, cellular transmissions, and all forms of radiation, in matter, dark matter, antimatter, energy, space, time, and all alternate realities, mind control, non-beneficial interdimensional beings, earthbound tricksters, extraterrestrials, artificial intelligence, subliminal messages, hypnosis and posthypnotic suggestions in all forms, parasites, viruses, non-beneficial bacteria, emotional charges, cords, attachments, implants, hooks, entities, and thought forms, seen or unseen, cloaked or uncloaked, in conscious, subconscious, and all altered states of consciousness, even if they are changing frequencies and dimensions, simultaneously, in matter, dark matter, antimatter, energy, space, time, and all alternate

realities. We are moving everything into the containment orb at the count of 10.

1, 2, 3, 4, 5, 6, 7, 8, 9, 10 - Increasing the cohesion to the 987th Fibonacci number.

We are clearing all imprints, echoes, residuals, energetic tattoos associated with what we just cleared, simultaneously, in matter, dark matter, antimatter, energy, space, time, and all alternate realities. We are moving everything into the containment orb at the count of 10.

1, 2, 3, 4, 5, 6, 7, 8, 9, 10 - Increasing the cohesion to the 987th Fibonacci number.

◓ (Projecting) We are sealing the containment orb.

◒ (Extracting) Sending it to the Central Sun.

And so it is, and so it is, and so it is.

EVENTS

◗ (Projecting) We are placing _____(Event Name/Location) in an orb with mirrors facing in and mirrors facing out, the Sirius B Council on the outside, Archangels Raphael, Uriel, Gabriel, and Michael at the four cardinal points.

We are placing a containment orb to the right of the main orb with mirrors facing in and mirrors facing out, the Sirius B Council on the outside, Archangels Raphael, Uriel, Gabriel, and Michael at the four cardinal points.

We invoke all the Ascended Masters and Angelic Beings of the Universe, to go up as a conduit through the Galactic Core, Central Sun, Secret Sun, Platinum Sun, into conscious, subconscious, and all altered states of consciousness, and come down into _____ (Event Name/Location).

◖ (Extracting) We are clearing _____(Event Name/Location), The staff, security, all attendees, and others involved in the production of the event, and everything else, including furniture, fixtures, appliances, personal property, and the ethers, from the manifest to the unmanifest, from particle to wave, transmuting to a neutral energy. Clearing all EMF energy fluctuations from solar flares and geomagnetic storms, cellular transmissions, and all forms of radiation, in matter, dark matter, antimatter, energy, space, time, and all alternate realities, mind control, non-beneficial interdimensional beings, earthbound tricksters, extraterrestrials, artificial intelligence, subliminal messages, hypnosis and posthypnotic suggestions in all forms, parasites, viruses, non-beneficial bacteria, collective-consciousness fear, anxiety, trauma, emotional charges, cords, attachments, implants, hooks, entities, and thought forms, seen or unseen, cloaked or uncloaked, in conscious, subconscious, and all altered states of consciousness, even if they are changing frequencies and dimensions, simultaneously, in matter, dark matter, antimatter,

energy, space, time, and all alternate realities. We are moving everything into the containment orb at the count of 10.

1, 2, 3, 4, 5, 6, 7, 8, 9, 10 - Increasing the cohesion to the 987th Fibonacci number.

We are clearing all imprints, echoes, residuals, energetic tattoos associated with what we just cleared, simultaneously, in matter, dark matter, antimatter, energy, space, time, and all alternate realities. We are moving everything into the containment orb at the count of 10.

1, 2, 3, 4, 5, 6, 7, 8, 9, 10 - Increasing the cohesion to the 987th Fibonacci number.

◯ (Projecting) We are sealing the containment orb.

◯ (Extracting) Sending it to the Central Sun.

And so it is, and so it is, and so it is.

HOME RESIDENCE

☾ (Projecting) We are placing an orb around _____(Location) with mirrors facing in and mirrors facing out, the Sirius B Council on the outside, Archangels Raphael, Uriel, Gabriel, and Michael at the four cardinal points.

We are placing a containment orb to the right of the main orb with mirrors facing in and mirrors facing out, the Sirius B Council on the outside, Archangels Raphael, Uriel, Gabriel, and Michael at the four cardinal points.

We invoke all the Ascended Masters and Angelic Beings of the Universe, to go up as a conduit through the Galactic Core, Central Sun, Secret Sun, Platinum Sun, into conscious, subconscious, and all altered states of consciousness, and come down into _____ (Location).

☾ (Extracting) We are clearing _____(Location) and all furniture, fixtures, appliances, personal property, children, adults, plants, and any pets in the home, the ethers, the ground below, the air above, from the manifest to the unmanifest, from particle to wave, transmuting to a neutral energy. Clearing all EMF energy fluctuations from solar flares and geomagnetic storms, cellular transmissions, and all forms of radiation, in matter, dark matter, antimatter, energy, space, time, and all alternate realities, mind control, non-beneficial interdimensional beings, earthbound tricksters, extraterrestrials, artificial intelligence, subliminal messages, hypnosis and posthypnotic suggestions in all forms, parasites, viruses, non-beneficial bacteria, collective-consciousness fear, anxiety, trauma, emotional charges, cords, attachments, implants, hooks, entities, and thought forms, seen or unseen, cloaked or uncloaked, in conscious, subconscious, and all altered states of consciousness, even if they are changing frequencies and dimensions, simultaneously, in matter,

dark matter, antimatter, energy, space, time, and all alternate realities. We are moving everything into the containment orb at the count of 10.

1, 2, 3, 4, 5, 6, 7, 8, 9, 10 - Increasing the cohesion to the 987th Fibonacci number.

We are clearing all imprints, echoes, residuals, energetic tattoos associated with what we just cleared, simultaneously, in matter, dark matter, antimatter, energy, space, time, and all alternate realities. We are moving everything into the containment orb at the count of 10.

1, 2, 3, 4, 5, 6, 7, 8, 9, 10 - Increasing the cohesion to the 987th Fibonacci number.

☌ (Projecting) We are sealing the containment orb.

☊ (Extracting) Sending it to the Central Sun.

And so it is, and so it is, and so it is.

HOTELS, MOTELS, TIMESHARES AND RENTALS

↷ (Projecting) We are placing _____(Name and Address) including the ground below, air above and any parking areas in an orb with mirrors facing in and mirrors facing out, the Sirius B Council on the outside, Archangels Raphael, Uriel, Gabriel, and Michael at the four cardinal points.

We are placing a containment orb to the right of the main orb with mirrors facing in and mirrors facing out, the Sirius B Council on the outside, Archangels Raphael, Uriel, Gabriel, and Michael at the four cardinal points.

We are invoking all the Ascended Masters and Angelic Beings of the Universe, to go up as a conduit through the Galactic Core, Central Sun, Secret Sun, Platinum Sun, into conscious, subconscious, and all altered states of consciousness, and down into _____ (Name and Address).

↶ (Extracting) We are clearing _____(Name and Address) all furniture, fixtures, appliances, elevators, public common areas, business centers, spas, and recreational facilities including jacuzzis, swimming pools, hot tubs, saunas, steam rooms, and personal property of trauma or negative energy infused in the property and the ethers, from the manifest to the unmanifest, from particle to wave, transmuting to a neutral energy. Clearing all EMF energy fluctuations from solar flares and geomagnetic storms, cellular transmissions, and all forms of radiation, in matter, dark matter, antimatter, energy, space, time, and all alternate realities, mind control, non-beneficial interdimensional beings, earthbound tricksters, extraterrestrials, artificial intelligence, subliminal messages, hypnosis and posthypnotic suggestions in all forms, parasites, viruses, non-beneficial bacteria, collective-consciousness fear, anxiety, trauma, emotional charges, cords, attachments, implants, hooks, entities, and thought forms, seen or unseen, cloaked or uncloaked, in conscious, subconscious, and all altered states of consciousness, even if they are changing frequencies and dimensions, simultaneously, in matter, dark matter, antimatter, energy, space, time, and all alternate realities. We are moving everything into the containment orb at the count of 10.

1, 2, 3, 4, 5, 6, 7, 8, 9, 10 - Increasing the cohesion to the 987th Fibonacci number.

We are clearing all imprints, echoes, residuals, energetic tattoos associated with what we just cleared, simultaneously, in matter, dark matter, antimatter, energy, space, time, and all alternate realities. We are moving everything into the containment orb at the count of 10.

1, 2, 3, 4, 5, 6, 7, 8, 9, 10 - Increasing the cohesion to the 987th Fibonacci number.

☽ (Projecting) We are sealing the containment orb.

☾ (Extracting) Sending it to the Central Sun.

And so it is, and so it is, and so it is.

HOTEL ROOM

☽ (Projecting) We are placing an orb around _____(Room Number/Name of Hotel) with mirrors facing in and mirrors facing out, the Sirius B Council on the outside, Archangels Raphael, Uriel, Gabriel, and Michael at the four cardinal points.

We are placing a containment orb to the right of the main orb with mirrors facing in and mirrors facing out, the Sirius B Council on the outside, Archangels Raphael, Uriel, Gabriel, and Michael at the four cardinal points.

We invoke all the Ascended Masters and Angelic Beings of the Universe, to go up as a conduit, through the Galactic Core, Central Sun, Secret Sun, Platinum Sun, into conscious, subconscious, and all altered states of consciousness, and come down into _____ (Room Number/Name of Hotel).

☽ (Extracting) We are clearing _____(Room Number/Name of Hotel), all furniture, fixtures, appliances, and personal property, zero pointing the energy in the room, from the manifest to the unmanifest, from particle to wave, transmuting to a neutral energy. Clearing all EMF energy fluctuations from solar flares and geomagnetic storms, cellular transmissions, and all forms of radiation, in matter, dark matter, antimatter, energy, space, time, and all alternate realities, mind control, non-beneficial interdimensional beings, earthbound tricksters, extraterrestrials, artificial intelligence, subliminal messages, hypnosis and posthypnotic suggestions in all forms, parasites, viruses, non-beneficial bacteria, collective-consciousness fear, anxiety, trauma, emotional charges, cords, attachments, implants, hooks, entities, and thought forms, seen or unseen, cloaked or uncloaked, in conscious, subconscious, and all altered states of consciousness, even if they are changing frequencies and dimensions, simultaneously, in matter, dark matter, antimatter, energy, space, time, and all alternate realities. We are moving everything into the containment orb at the count of 10.

1, 2, 3, 4, 5, 6, 7, 8, 9, 10 - Increasing the cohesion to the 987th Fibonacci number.

We are clearing all imprints, echoes, residuals, energetic tattoos associated with what we just cleared, simultaneously, in matter, dark matter, antimatter, energy, space, time, and all alternate realities. We are moving everything into the containment orb at the count of 10.

1, 2, 3, 4, 5, 6, 7, 8, 9, 10 - Increasing the cohesion to the 987th Fibonacci number.

⟳ (Projecting) We are sealing the containment orb.

⟲ (Extracting) Sending it to the Central Sun.

And so it is, and so it is, and so it is.

JOB INTERVIEW

☽ (Projecting) We are placing the _____(Location of Interview) in an orb with mirrors facing in and mirrors facing out, the Sirius B Council on the outside, Archangels Raphael, Uriel, Gabriel, and Michael at the four cardinal points.

We are placing a containment orb to the right of the main orb with mirrors facing in and mirrors facing out, the Sirius B Council on the outside, Archangels Raphael, Uriel, Gabriel, and Michael at the four cardinal points.

We invoke all the Ascended Masters and Angelic Beings of the Universe, to go up as a conduit, through the Galactic Core, Central Sun, Secret Sun, Platinum Sun, into conscious, subconscious, and all altered states of consciousness, and come down into _____ (Interviewer) and _____(Person being Interviewed).

☽ (Extracting) We are clearing the _____(Interviewer) and _____(Person Being Interviewed), from the manifest to the unmanifest, from particle to wave, transmuting to a neutral energy. Clearing all EMF energy fluctuations from solar flares and geomagnetic storms, cellular transmissions, and all forms of radiation, in matter, dark matter, antimatter, energy, space, time, and all alternate realities, mind control, non-beneficial interdimensional beings, earthbound tricksters, extraterrestrials, artificial intelligence, subliminal messages, hypnosis and posthypnotic suggestions in all forms, parasites, viruses, non-beneficial bacteria, collective-consciousness fear, anxiety, trauma, emotional charges, cords, attachments, implants, hooks, entities, and thought forms, seen or unseen, cloaked or uncloaked, in conscious, subconscious, and all altered states of consciousness, even if they are changing frequencies and dimensions, simultaneously, in matter, dark matter, antimatter, energy, space, time, and all alternate realities. We are moving everything into the containment orb at the count of 10.

1, 2, 3, 4, 5, 6, 7, 8, 9, 10 - Increasing the cohesion to the 987th Fibonacci number.

We are clearing all imprints, echoes, residuals, energetic tattoos associated with what we just cleared, simultaneously, in matter, dark matter, antimatter, energy, space, time, and all alternate realities. We are moving everything into the containment orb at the count of 10.

1, 2, 3, 4, 5, 6, 7, 8, 9, 10 - Increasing the cohesion to the 987th Fibonacci number.

↷ (Projecting) We are sealing the containment orb.

↶ (Extracting) Sending it to the Central Sun.

And so it is, and so it is, and so it is.

LOCATION

◗ (Projecting) We are placing _____(Location), including the ground below, the air above and any parking areas, in an orb with mirrors facing in and mirrors facing out, the Sirius B Council on the outside, Archangels Raphael, Uriel, Gabriel, and Michael at the four cardinal points.

We are placing a containment orb to the right of the main orb with mirrors facing in and mirrors facing out, the Sirius B Council on the outside, Archangels Raphael, Uriel, Gabriel, and Michael at the four cardinal points.

We are invoking all the Ascended Masters and Angelic Beings of the Universe, to go up as a conduit, through the Galactic Core, Central Sun, Secret Sun, Platinum Sun, into conscious, subconscious, and all altered states of consciousness, and come down into _____ (Location).

◖ (Extracting) We are clearing _____(Location) and all furniture, fixtures, appliances, personal property, and the ethers, from the manifest to the unmanifest, from particle to wave, transmuting to a neutral energy. Clearing all EMF energy fluctuations from solar flares and geomagnetic storms, cellular transmissions, and all forms of radiation, in matter, dark matter, antimatter, energy, space, time, and all alternate realities, mind control, non-beneficial interdimensional beings, earthbound tricksters, extraterrestrials, artificial intelligence, subliminal messages, hypnosis and posthypnotic suggestions in all forms, parasites, viruses, non-beneficial bacteria, collective-consciousness fear, anxiety, trauma, emotional charges, cords, attachments, implants, hooks, entities, and thought forms, seen or unseen, cloaked or uncloaked, in conscious, subconscious, and all altered states of consciousness, even if they are changing frequencies and dimensions, simultaneously, in matter, dark matter, antimatter, energy, space, time, and all alternate realities. We are moving everything into the containment orb at the count of 10.

1, 2, 3, 4, 5, 6, 7, 8, 9, 10 - Increasing the cohesion to the 987th Fibonacci number.

We are clearing all imprints, echoes, residuals, energetic tattoos associated with what we just cleared, simultaneously, in matter, dark matter, antimatter, energy, space, time, and all alternate realities. We are moving everything into the containment orb at the count of 10.

1, 2, 3, 4, 5, 6, 7, 8, 9, 10 - Increasing the cohesion to the 987th Fibonacci number.

◠➔ (Projecting) We are sealing the containment orb.

◠ (Extracting) Sending it to the Central Sun.

And so it is, and so it is, and so it is.

OFFICE/BUSINESS

◗ (Projecting) We are placing _____(Location/Office or Business) in an orb with mirrors facing in and mirrors facing out, the Sirius B Council on the outside, Archangels Raphael, Uriel, Gabriel, and Michael at the four cardinal points.

We are placing a containment orb to the right of the main orb with mirrors facing in and mirrors facing out, the Sirius B Council on the outside, Archangels Raphael, Uriel, Gabriel, and Michael at the four cardinal points.

We invoke all the Ascended Masters and Angelic Beings of the Universe, to go up as a conduit, through the Galactic Core, Central Sun, Secret Sun, Platinum Sun, into conscious, subconscious, and all altered states of consciousness, and come down into _____ (Location/Office or Business).

◖ (Extracting) We are clearing _____(Location/Office or Business) of conflicts or negative energy between the people who work there and the customers; we are clearing all furniture, fixtures, appliances, personal property, and the ethers, from the manifest to the unmanifest, from particle to wave, transmuting to a neutral energy. Clearing all EMF energy fluctuations from solar flares and geomagnetic storms, cellular transmissions, and all forms of radiation, in matter, dark matter, antimatter, energy, space, time, and all alternate realities, mind control, non-beneficial interdimensional beings, earthbound tricksters, extraterrestrials, artificial intelligence, subliminal messages, hypnosis and posthypnotic suggestions in all forms, parasites, viruses, non-beneficial bacteria, collective-consciousness fear, anxiety, trauma, emotional charges, cords, attachments, implants, hooks, entities, and thought forms, seen or unseen, cloaked or uncloaked, in conscious, subconscious, and all altered states of consciousness, even if they are changing frequencies and dimensions, simultaneously, in matter, dark matter, antimatter,

energy, space, time, and all alternate realities. We are moving everything into the containment orb at the count of 10.

1, 2, 3, 4, 5, 6, 7, 8, 9, 10 - Increasing the cohesion to the 987th Fibonacci number.

We are clearing all imprints, echoes, residuals, energetic tattoos associated with what we just cleared, simultaneously, in matter, dark matter, antimatter, energy, space, time, and all alternate realities. We are moving everything into the containment orb at the count of 10.

1, 2, 3, 4, 5, 6, 7, 8, 9, 10 - Increasing the cohesion to the 987th Fibonacci number.

(Projecting) We are sealing the containment orb.

(Extracting) Sending it to the Central Sun.

(Projecting) We invoke all the Ascended Masters and Angelic Beings of the Universe to go up as a conduit, through the Galactic Core, Central Sun, Secret Sun, Platinum Sun, in conscious, subconscious, and all altered states of consciousness. We are opening a portal of Galactic light into _____(Location/Office or Business) and we are raising the vibration and increasing the frequency of _____(Location/Office or Business) to the frequency of Galactic light code with a continuous loop until such time it is requested to be stopped.

And so it is, and so it is, and so it is.

PREVIOUS RESIDENCE/ WORK LOCATION

◑ (Projecting) We are placing _____(Previous Location), including the ground below, air above, and any parking areas, in an orb with mirrors facing in and mirrors facing out, the Sirius B Council on the outside, Archangels Raphael, Uriel, Gabriel, and Michael at the four cardinal points.

We are placing a containment orb to the right of the main orb with mirrors facing in and mirrors facing out, the Sirius B Council on the outside, Archangels Raphael, Uriel, Gabriel, and Michael at the four cardinal points.

We invoke all the Ascended Masters and Angelic Beings of the Universe, to go up as a conduit, through the Galactic Core, Central Sun, Secret Sun, Platinum Sun, into conscious, subconscious, and all altered states of consciousness, and come down into _____ (Previous Location).

◔ (Extracting) We are clearing _____(Previous Location) of all energy associated with _____(Name) so there is no current or future connections with that location, from the manifest to the unmanifest, from particle to wave, transmuting to a neutral energy, We are clearing all EMF energy fluctuations from solar flares and geomagnetic storms, cellular transmissions, and all forms of radiation, in matter, dark matter, antimatter, energy, space, time, and all alternate realities, mind control, non-beneficial interdimensional beings, earthbound tricksters, extraterrestrials, artificial intelligence, subliminal messages, hypnosis and posthypnotic suggestions in all forms, parasites, viruses, non-beneficial bacteria, collective-consciousness fear, anxiety, trauma, emotional charges, cords, attachments, implants, hooks, entities, and thought forms, seen or unseen, cloaked or uncloaked, in conscious, subconscious, and all altered states of consciousness, even if they are changing frequencies and dimensions, simultaneously, in matter, dark matter, antimatter, energy, space, time, and all alternate realities. We are moving everything into the containment orb at the count of 10.

1, 2, 3, 4, 5, 6, 7, 8, 9, 10 - Increasing the cohesion to the 987th Fibonacci number.

We are clearing all imprints, echoes, residuals, energetic tattoos associated with what we just cleared, simultaneously, in matter, dark matter, antimatter, energy, space, time, and all alternate realities. We are moving everything into the containment orb at the count of 10.

1, 2, 3, 4, 5, 6, 7, 8, 9, 10 - Increasing the cohesion to the 987th Fibonacci number.

(Projecting) We are sealing the containment orb.

(Extracting) Sending it to the Central Sun.

And so it is, and so it is, and so it is.

RESTAURANT

☽ (Projecting) We are placing _____(Name of Restaurant) in an orb with mirrors facing in and mirrors facing out, the Sirius B Council on the outside, Archangels Raphael, Uriel, Gabriel, and Michael at the four cardinal points.

We are placing a containment orb to the right of the main orb with mirrors facing in and mirrors facing out, the Sirius B Council on the outside, Archangels Raphael, Uriel, Gabriel, and Michael at the four cardinal points.

We invoke all the Ascended Masters and Angelic Beings of the Universe, to go up as a conduit, through the Galactic Core, Central Sun, Secret Sun, Platinum Sun, into conscious, subconscious, and all altered states of consciousness, and come down into _____ (Name of Restaurant).

☾ (Extracting) We are clearing the restaurant of conflicts and negative energy between the people who work there and the customers; we are clearing the restaurant front of house, decor, furniture, fixtures, and all surfaces of the building, kitchen, storerooms, walk-in and reach-in refrigeration, dry storage, food prep, cooking line, waitstaff pickup area, and management offices, from the manifest to the unmanifest, from particle to wave, transmuting to a neutral energy. Clearing all EMF energy fluctuations from solar flares and geomagnetic storms, cellular transmissions, and all forms of radiation, in matter, dark matter, antimatter, energy, space, time, and all alternate realities, mind control, non-beneficial interdimensional beings, earthbound tricksters, extraterrestrials, artificial intelligence, subliminal messages, hypnosis and posthypnotic suggestions in all forms, parasites, viruses, non-beneficial bacteria, collective-consciousness fear, anxiety, trauma, emotional charges, cords, attachments, alcohol, drugs and all other implants, hooks, entities, and thought forms, seen or unseen, cloaked or uncloaked, in conscious, subconscious, and all altered states of consciousness, even

if they are changing frequencies and dimensions, simultaneously, in matter, dark matter, antimatter, energy, space, time, and all alternate realities. We are moving everything into the containment orb at the count of 10.

1, 2, 3, 4, 5, 6, 7, 8, 9, 10 - Increasing the cohesion to the 987th Fibonacci number.

We are clearing all imprints, echoes, residuals, energetic tattoos associated with what we just cleared, simultaneously, in matter, dark matter, antimatter, energy, space, time, and all alternate realities into the containment orb at the count of 10.

1, 2, 3, 4, 5, 6, 7, 8, 9, 10 - Increasing the cohesion to the 987th Fibonacci number.

↻ (Projecting) We are sealing the containment orb.

↺ (Extracting) Sending it to the Central Sun.

And so it is, and so it is, and so it is.

CHAPTER 3

ELEMENTAL TRANSMUTATION

SEVERE WEATHER MITIGATION

☽ (Projecting) We are placing 987 trillion holographic duplicates of _____(Name of Storm) all across the universe, 987 trillion holographic mirrored orbs, triangles, merkabas, pyramids, and Christ chambers over, under and around _____(Name of Storm). We are cloaking and making _____(Name of Storm) holographically invisible in the spirit realms on a fractal, atomic and cellular level, in matter, dark matter, antimatter, energy, space, time, and all alternate realities.

We are placing _____(Name of Storm) in an orb with mirrors facing in and mirrors facing out, the Sirius B Council on the outside, Archangels Raphael, Uriel, Gabriel, and Michael at the four cardinal points.

We are placing a containment orb to the right of the main orb with mirrors facing in and mirrors facing out, the Sirius B Council on the outside, Archangels Raphael, Uriel, Gabriel, and Michael at the four cardinal points.

We invoke all the Ascended Masters and Angelic Beings of the Universe to go up as a conduit, through the Galactic Core, Central Sun, Secret Sun, Platinum Sun, into conscious, subconscious, and all altered states of consciousness, and come down into _____ (Name of Storm).

☾ (Extracting) We now encapsulate the eye of _____(Name of Storm), from the manifest to the unmanifest, from particle to wave, transmuting to a neutral energy, seen or unseen, cloaked or uncloaked, even if _____(Name of Storm) is changing frequencies and dimensions, simultaneously, in matter, dark matter, antimatter, energy, space, time, and all alternate realities We are moving the encapsulated eye of _____(Name of Storm) into the containment orb at the count of 10.

1, 2, 3, 4, 5, 6, 7, 8, 9, 10 - Increasing the cohesion to the 987th Fibonacci number.

We are clearing all imprints, echoes, residuals, energetic tattoos associated with what we just cleared, simultaneously, in matter, dark matter, antimatter, energy, space, time, and all alternate realities. We are moving everything into the containment orb at the count of 10.

1, 2, 3, 4, 5, 6, 7, 8, 9, 10 - Increasing the cohesion to the 987th Fibonacci number.

◗ (Projecting) We are sealing the containment orb.

◖ (Extracting) Sending it to the Central Sun.

And so it is, and so it is, and so it is.

STRUCTURED WATER

↷ (Projecting) We are placing the water in an orb with mirrors facing in and mirrors facing out, the Sirius B Council on the outside, Archangels Raphael, Uriel, Gabriel, and Michael at the four cardinal points.

We are placing a containment orb to the right of the main orb with mirrors facing in and mirrors facing out, the Sirius B Council on the outside, Archangels Raphael, Uriel, Gabriel, and Michael at the four cardinal points.

We invoke all the Ascended Masters and Angelic Beings of the Universe to go up as a conduit, through the Galactic Core, Central Sun, Secret Sun, Platinum Sun, into conscious, subconscious, and all altered states of consciousness, and come down in the water.

↶ (Extracting) We are clearing the water of all mineral impurities and imbalances, from the manifest to the unmanifest, from particle to wave, transmuting to a neutral energy. Clearing all EMF energy fluctuations from solar flares and geomagnetic storms, cellular transmissions, and all forms of radiation, in matter, dark matter, antimatter, energy, space, time, and all alternate realities, mind control, non-beneficial interdimensional beings, earthbound tricksters, extraterrestrials, artificial intelligence, subliminal messages, hypnosis and posthypnotic suggestions in all forms, parasites, viruses, non-beneficial bacteria, collective-consciousness fear, anxiety, trauma, emotional charges, cords, attachments, implants, hooks, entities, and thought forms, seen or unseen, cloaked or uncloaked, in conscious, subconscious, and all altered states of consciousness, even if they are changing frequencies and dimensions, simultaneously, in matter, dark matter, antimatter, energy, space, time, and all alternate realities. We are moving everything into the containment orb at the count of 10.

1, 2, 3, 4, 5, 6, 7, 8, 9, 10 - Increasing the cohesion to the 987th Fibonacci number.

We are clearing all imprints, echoes, residuals, energetic tattoos associated with what we just cleared, simultaneously, in matter, dark matter, antimatter, energy, space, time, and all alternate realities into the containment orb at the count of 10.

1, 2, 3, 4, 5, 6, 7, 8, 9, 10 - Increasing the cohesion to the 987th Fibonacci number.

↷ (Projecting) We are sealing the containment orb.

↶ (Extracting) Sending it to the Central Sun.

↷ (Projecting) We invoke all the Ascended Masters and Angelic Beings of the Universe to go up as a conduit, through the Galactic Core, Central Sun, Secret Sun, Platinum Sun, into conscious, subconscious, and all altered states of consciousness, and raise the vibration of the water to the highest galactic frequency at which it can vibrate.

And so it is, and so it is, and so it is.

WINE

◗ (Projecting) We are placing the wine in an orb with mirrors facing in and mirrors facing out, the Sirius B Council on the outside, Archangels Raphael, Uriel, Gabriel, and Michael at the four cardinal points.

We are placing a containment orb to the right of the main orb with mirrors facing in and mirrors facing out, the Sirius B Council on the outside, Archangels Raphael, Uriel, Gabriel, and Michael at the four cardinal points.

We invoke all the Ascended Masters and Angelic Beings of the universe to go up as a conduit, through the Galactic Core, Central Sun, Secret Sun, Platinum Sun into conscious, subconscious, and all altered states of consciousness, and then come down into the wine.

◖ (Extracting) We are clearing the wine of all impurities, issues with too much or too little sunshine or rain, temperature fluctuations, and other issues which had prevented this wine from achieving its full potential, from the manifest to the unmanifest, from particle to wave, transmuting to a neutral energy. Clearing all EMF energy fluctuations from solar flares and geomagnetic storms, cellular transmissions, and all forms of radiation, in matter, dark matter, antimatter, energy, space, time, and all alternate realities, mind control, non-beneficial interdimensional beings, earthbound trick-sters, extraterrestrials, artificial intelligence, subliminal messages, hypnosis and posthypnotic suggestions in all forms, parasites, viruses, non-beneficial bacteria, collective-consciousness fear, anxiety, trauma, emotional charges, cords, attachments, implants, hooks, entities, and thought forms, seen or unseen, cloaked or uncloaked, in conscious, subconscious, and all altered states of consciousness, even if they are changing frequencies and dimensions, simultaneously, in matter, dark matter, antimatter, energy, space, time, and all alternate realities. We are moving everything into the containment orb at the count of 10.

1, 2, 3, 4, 5, 6, 7, 8, 9, 10 - Increasing the cohesion to the 987th Fibonacci number.

We are clearing all imprints, echoes, residuals, energetic tattoos associated with what we just cleared, simultaneously, in matter, dark matter, antimatter, energy, space, time, and all alternate realities into the containment orb at the count of 10.

1, 2, 3, 4, 5, 6, 7, 8, 9, 10 - Increasing the cohesion to the 987th Fibonacci number.

(Projecting) We are sealing the containment orb.

(Extracting) Sending it to the Central Sun.

(Projecting) We invoke all the Ascended Masters and Angelic Beings of the Universe to go up as a conduit, through the Galactic Core, Central Sun, Secret Sun, Platinum Sun, into conscious, subconscious, and all altered states of consciousness, and come down to energetically perfect the wine to its full quality potential and raise the vibration of the wine to the highest frequency at which it can vibrate.

And so it is, and so it is, and so it is.

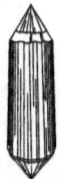

CHAPTER 4

BROKEN HEARTS

ABANDONMENT

◯ (Projecting) We are placing _____(Name) in an orb with mirrors facing in and mirrors facing out, the Sirius B Council on the outside, Archangels Raphael, Uriel, Gabriel, and Michael at the four cardinal points.

We are placing a containment orb to the right of the main orb with mirrors facing in and mirrors facing out, the Sirius B Council on the outside, Archangels Raphael, Uriel, Gabriel, and Michael at the four cardinal points.

We invoke all the Ascended Masters and Angelic Beings of the Universe to go up as a conduit, through the Galactic Core, Central Sun, Secret Sun, Platinum Sun, into conscious, subconscious, and all altered states of consciousness, and come down into _____(Name).

◯ (Extracting) We are clearing _____(Name) from the abandonment, anxiety, trauma, feelings of a broken heart, betrayal, deception, breach of trust, shock, and fear from the cellular DNA throughout _____(Name) entire physical body and auric field, from the manifest to the unmanifest, from particle to wave, transmuting to a neutral energy. Clearing all EMF energy fluctuations from solar flares and geomagnetic storms, cellular transmissions, and all forms of radiation, in matter, dark matter, antimatter, energy, space, time, and all alternate realities, mind control, non-beneficial interdimensional beings, earthbound tricksters, extraterrestrials, artificial intelligence, subliminal messages, hypnosis and posthypnotic suggestions in all forms, parasites, viruses, non-beneficial bacteria, collective-consciousness fear, anxiety, trauma, emotional charges, cords, attachments, implants, hooks, entities, and thought forms, seen or unseen, cloaked or uncloaked, in conscious, subconscious, and all altered states of consciousness, even if they are changing frequencies and dimensions, simultaneously, in matter, dark matter, antimatter, energy, space, time, and alternative realities.

We are moving everything into the containment orb at the count of 10.

1, 2, 3, 4, 5, 6, 7, 8, 9, 10 – Increasing the cohesion to the 987th Fibonacci number.

We are clearing all imprints, echoes, residuals, energetic tattoos associated with what we just cleared, simultaneously, in matter, dark matter, antimatter, energy, space, time, and all alternate realities. We are moving everything into the containment orb at the count of 10.

1, 2, 3, 4, 5, 6, 7, 8, 9, 10 – Increasing the cohesion to the 987th Fibonacci number

☽ (Projecting) We are sealing the containment orb.

☾ (Extracting) Sending it to the Central Sun.

And so it is, and so it is, and so it is.

EARTHBOUND SPIRITS

↻ (Projecting) We invoke all the Ascended Masters and Angelic Beings of the Universe to go up as a conduit, through the Galactic Core, Central Sun, Secret Sun, Platinum Sun, into conscious, subconscious, and all altered states of consciousness, to create a large column of glittering shimmering galactic light from the Galactic Core to _____(Name), and we call in from the other side disincarnate close, immediate family and pets to assist _____(Name) and invoke all the Ascended Masters and Angelic Beings of the Universe to go up as a conduit, into conscious, subconscious, and all altered states of consciousness to assist the disincarnate family members and pets to help _____(Name) to cross into the light at the count of 10.

1, 2, 3, 4, 5, 6, 7, 8, 9, 10 - Increasing the cohesion to the 987th Fibonacci number.

And so it is, and so it is, and so it is.

GRIEVING AFTER LOSS/ SUICIDE

☽ (Projecting) We are placing _____(Name of the Person Grieving) in an orb with mirrors facing in and mirrors facing out, the Sirius B Council on the outside, Archangels Raphael, Uriel, Gabriel, and Michael at the four cardinal points.

We are placing a containment orb to the right of the main orb with mirrors facing in and mirrors facing out, the Sirius B Council on the outside, Archangels Raphael, Uriel, Gabriel, and Michael at the four cardinal points.

We invoke all the Ascended Masters and Angelic Beings of the Universe to go up as a conduit, through the Galactic Core, Central Sun, Secret Sun, Platinum Sun, into conscious, subconscious, and all altered states of consciousness and come down into _____ (Name of the Person Grieving).

☾ (Extracting) We are clearing _____(Name of the Person Grieving) of the profound sadness, grief, sense of loss, and emotional charges associated with the loss of _____(Name of the Person Who Transitioned), from the manifest to the unmanifest, from particle to wave, transmuting to a neutral energy and invoke the Ascended Masters and Angelic beings of the Universe to go up as a conduit, through the Galactic Core, Central Sun, Secret Sun, Platinum Sun, into conscious, subconscious, and all altered states of consciousness and come into _____(Name of the Person Grieving) clearing all emotional charges and collapsing the energy to zero point, seen or unseen, cloaked or uncloaked, even if they are changing frequencies and dimensions, simultaneously, in matter, dark matter, antimatter, energy, space, time, and all alternate realities. We are moving everything into the containment orb at the count of 10.

1, 2, 3, 4, 5, 6, 7, 8, 9, 10 - Increasing the cohesion to the 987th Fibonacci number.

We are clearing all imprints, echoes, residuals, energetic tattoos associated with what we just cleared, simultaneously, in matter, dark matter, antimatter, energy, space, time, and all alternate realities. We are moving everything into the containment orb at the count of 10.

1, 2, 3, 4, 5, 6, 7, 8, 9, 10 - Increasing the cohesion to the 987th Fibonacci number.

↻ (Projecting) We are sealing the containment orb.

↺ (Extracting) Sending it to the Central Sun.

And so it is, and so it is, and so it is.

HOMICIDE

☽ (Projecting) We are placing the physical location of the homicide in an orb with mirrors facing in and mirrors facing out, the Sirius B Council on the outside, Archangels Raphael, Uriel, Gabriel, and Michael at the four cardinal points.

We are placing a containment orb to the right of the main orb with mirrors facing in and mirrors facing out, the Sirius B Council on the outside, Archangels Raphael, Uriel, Gabriel, and Michael at the four cardinal points.

We invoke all the Ascended Masters and Angelic Beings of the Universe to go up as a conduit, through the Galactic Core, Central Sun, Secret Sun, Platinum Sun, into conscious, subconscious, and all altered states of consciousness at the physical location of the homicide.

☾ (Extracting) We are clearing _____(Name of Homicide Victim) and the location of the homicide from the shock, pain, grief, trauma, from the manifest to the unmanifest, from particle to wave, transmuting to a neutral energy, all emotional charges, cords, attachments, implants, hooks, entities, and thought forms, seen or unseen, cloaked or uncloaked, into conscious, subconscious, and all altered states of consciousness, even if they are changing frequencies and dimensions, simultaneously, in matter, dark matter, antimatter, energy, space, time, and all alternate realities. We are moving everything into the containment orb at the count of 10.

1, 2, 3, 4, 5, 6, 7, 8, 9, 10 - Increasing the cohesion to the 987th Fibonacci number.

We are clearing all imprints, echoes, residuals, energetic tattoos associated with what we just cleared, simultaneously, in matter, dark matter, antimatter, energy, space, time, and all alternate

realities. We are moving everything into the containment orb at the count of 10.

1, 2, 3, 4, 5, 6, 7, 8, 9, 10 - Increasing the cohesion to the 987th Fibonacci number.

◠ (Projecting) We are sealing the containment orb.

◠ (Extracting) Sending it to the Central Sun.

◠ (Projecting) We invoke all the Ascended Masters and Angelic Beings of the Universe to go up as a conduit, through the Galactic Core, Central Sun, Secret Sun, Platinum Sun, creating a large column of glittering, shimmering Galactic Light going into conscious, subconscious, and all altered states of consciousness into _____ (Name of Homicide Victim), and we invoke from the other side disincarnate close immediate family and pets to assist _____ (Name of Homicide Victim) and invoke all the Ascended Masters and Angelic Beings of the Universe to go up as a conduit through the Galactic Core, Central Sun, Secret Sun, Platinum Sun, in conscious, subconscious, and all altered states of consciousness, to assist the disincarnate family members and pets helping _____(Name of Homicide Victim) to cross into the light.

And so it is, and so it is, and so it is.

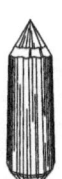

CHAPTER 5

HEALTH AND WELL BEING

BLOOD TRANSFUSIONS

☽ (Projecting) We are placing _____(Recipient of Blood Transfusion) and the donor blood on a horizontal podium, inside an orb with mirrors facing in and mirrors facing out, the Sirius B Council on the outside, Archangels Raphael, Uriel, Gabriel, and Michael at the four cardinal points.

We are placing a containment orb to the right of the main orb with mirrors facing in and mirrors facing out, the Sirius B Council on the outside, Archangels Raphael, Uriel, Gabriel, and Michael at the four cardinal points.

We invoke all the Ascended Masters and Angelic Beings of the Universe to go up as a conduit, through the Galactic Core, Central Sun, Secret Sun, Platinum Sun, into conscious, subconscious, and all altered states of consciousness and come down into _____ (Recipient of Blood Transfusion).

☽ (Extracting) We are clearing all imbalances between the vibration of the donated blood and the blood recipient. We are merging the donated blood's DNA and genetic coding with the recipient's blood into one energy frequency representative of the soul of the blood recipient, from the manifest to the unmanifest, from particle to wave, transmuting to a neutral energy. Clearing all EMF energy fluctuations from solar flares and geomagnetic storms, cellular transmissions, and all forms of radiation, in matter, dark matter, anti-matter, energy, space, time, and all alternate realities, mind control, non-beneficial interdimensional beings, earthbound tricksters, extraterrestrials, artificial intelligence, subliminal messages, hypnosis and posthypnotic suggestions in all forms, parasites, viruses, non-beneficial bacteria, collective-consciousness fear, anxiety, trauma in all forms, emotional charges, cords, attachments, implants, hooks, entities, and thought forms, seen or unseen, cloaked or uncloaked, in conscious, subconscious, and all altered states of consciousness, even if they are changing frequencies and dimensions, between

_____(Recipient of Blood Transfusion) and the donor blood, simultaneously, in matter, dark matter, antimatter, energy, space, time, and all alternate realities. We are moving everything into the containment orb at the count of 10.

1, 2, 3, 4, 5, 6, 7, 8, 9, 10 - Increasing the cohesion to the 987th Fibonacci number.

We are clearing all imprints, echoes, residuals, energetic tattoos associated with what we just cleared, simultaneously, in matter, dark matter, antimatter, energy, space, time, and all alternate realities. We are moving everything into the containment orb at the count of 10.

1, 2, 3, 4, 5, 6, 7, 8, 9, 10 - Increasing the cohesion to the 987th Fibonacci number.

◗ (Projecting) We are sealing the containment orb.

◖ (Extracting) Sending it to the Central Sun.

◗ (Projecting) We invoke all the Ascended Masters and Angelic Beings of the Universe to go up as a conduit, through the Galactic Core, Central Sun, Secret Sun, Platinum Sun, into conscious, subconscious, and all altered states of consciousness, and ask them to holographically equalize the donated blood to the same vibration, frequency and dimension at which the recipient's blood presently vibrates, and to holographically bind and transmute the donated blood's DNA and genetic coding to the DNA and genetic coding of the recipient, anchoring the holographic higher self of the blood recipient into the physical body and fully grounding into the crystal core of the Mother.

And so it is, and so it is, and so it is.

BONE MARROW

↻ (Projecting) We are placing _____(Name) in an orb with mirrors facing in and mirrors facing out, the Sirius B Council on the outside, Archangels Raphael, Uriel, Gabriel, and Michael at the four cardinal points.

We invoke all the Ascended Masters and Angelic Beings of the Universe to go up as a conduit, through the Galactic Core, Central Sun, Secret Sun, Platinum Sun, into conscious, subconscious, and all altered states of consciousness, and down into _____(Name) and to holographically infuse sufficient bone marrow in all the bones throughout the body and to fully lubricate every bone so there are no dry areas in any bones throughout the entire body, anchoring the holographic higher self into the physical body and fully grounding into the crystal core of the Mother.

And so it is, and so it is, and so it is.

DOCTOR'S OFFICE

☽ (Projecting) We are placing _____(Doctor's Office) in an orb with mirrors facing in and mirrors facing out, the Sirius B Council on the outside, Archangels Raphael, Uriel, Gabriel, and Michael at the four cardinal points.

We are placing a containment orb to the right of the main orb with mirrors facing in and mirrors facing out, the Sirius B Council on the outside, Archangels Raphael, Uriel, Gabriel, and Michael at the four cardinal points.

We invoke all the Ascended Masters and Angelic Beings of the Universe to go up as a conduit, through the Galactic Core, Central Sun, Secret Sun, Platinum Sun, into conscious, subconscious, and all altered states of consciousness and come down into _____ (Doctor's Office).

☾ (Extracting) We are clearing _____(Doctor's Office), all of the medical and administrative staff, patients, pharmaceutical, medical, diagnostic equipment reps and salespeople, including caterers in the doctor's office, as well as furniture, fixtures, appliances, medical instruments, devices, and medications, from the manifest to the unmanifest, from particle to wave, transmuting to a neutral energy. Clearing all EMF energy fluctuations from solar flares and geomagnetic storms, cellular transmissions, and all forms of radiation, in matter, dark matter, antimatter, energy, space, time, and all alternate realities, mind control, non-beneficial interdimensional beings, earthbound tricksters, extraterrestrials, artificial intelligence, subliminal messages, hypnosis and posthypnotic suggestions in all forms, parasites, viruses, non-beneficial bacteria, collective-consciousness fear, anxiety, trauma, emotional charges, cords, attachments, implants, hooks, entities, and thought forms, seen or unseen, cloaked or uncloaked, in conscious, subconscious, and all altered states of consciousness, even if they are changing frequencies and dimensions, simultaneously, in matter, dark matter, antimatter,

energy, space, time, and all alternate realities. We are moving everything into the containment orb at the count of 10.

1, 2, 3, 4, 5, 6, 7, 8, 9, 10 - Increasing the cohesion to the 987th Fibonacci number.

We are clearing all imprints, echoes, residuals, energetic tattoos associated with what we just cleared, simultaneously, in matter, dark matter, antimatter, energy, space, time, and all alternate realities. We are moving everything into the containment orb at the count of 10.

1, 2, 3, 4, 5, 6, 7, 8, 9, 10 - Increasing the cohesion to the 987th Fibonacci number.

◝ (Projecting) We are sealing the containment orb.

◜ (Extracting) Sending it to the Central Sun

And so it is, and so it is, and so it is.

HAIR MEMORY

☾ (Projecting) We are placing _____(Name) inside an orb with mirrors facing in and mirrors facing out, the Sirius B Council on the outside, Archangels Raphael, Uriel, Gabriel, and Michael at the four cardinal points.

We are placing a containment orb to the right of the main orb with mirrors facing in and mirrors facing out, the Sirius B Council on the outside, Archangels Raphael, Uriel, Gabriel, and Michael at the four cardinal points.

We invoke all the Ascended Masters and Angelic Beings of the Universe to go up as a conduit, through the Galactic Core, Central Sun, Secret Sun, Platinum Sun, into conscious, subconscious, and all altered states of consciousness, and come down into _____(Name).

☾ (Extracting) We are clearing all hair follicles and hair extensions (if any) of emotional charges, stored memory, imbalances, from the manifest to the unmanifest, from particle to wave, transmuting to a neutral energy. Clearing all EMF energy fluctuations from solar flares and geomagnetic storms, cellular transmissions, and all forms of radiation, in matter, dark matter, antimatter, energy, space, time, and all alternate realities, mind control, non-beneficial interdimensional beings, earthbound tricksters, extraterrestrials, artificial intelligence, subliminal messages, hypnosis and posthypnotic suggestions in all forms, parasites, viruses, non-beneficial bacteria, collective-consciousness fear, anxiety, trauma, emotional charges, cords, attachments, implants, hooks, entities, and thought forms, seen or unseen, cloaked or uncloaked, in conscious, subconscious, and all altered states of consciousness, even if they are changing frequencies and dimensions, simultaneously, in matter, dark matter, antimatter, energy, space, time, and all alternate realities. We are moving everything into the containment orb at the count of 10.

1, 2, 3, 4, 5, 6, 7, 8, 9, 10 - Increasing the cohesion to the 987th Fibonacci number.

We are clearing all imprints, echoes, residuals, energetic tattoos associated with what we just cleared, simultaneously, in matter, dark matter, antimatter, energy, space, time, and all alternate realities. We are moving everything into the containment orb at the count of 10.

1, 2, 3, 4, 5, 6, 7, 8, 9, 10 - Increasing the cohesion to the 987th Fibonacci number.

↷ (Projecting) We are sealing the containment orb.

↶ (Extracting) Sending it to the Central Sun.

↷ (Projecting) We invoke all the Ascended Masters and Angelic Beings of the Universe to go up as a conduit, through the Galactic Core, Central Sun, Secret Sun, Platinum Sun, into conscious, subconscious, and all altered states of consciousness, and radiate the hair follicles, including hair extentions, hairpieces and hair transplants to the same vibration, frequency and dimension at which _____ (Name) hair is currently vibrating, and to permanently transmute the memory in the hair follicles DNA and genetic coding to zero point, anchoring the holographic higher self into the physical body and fully grounding into the crystal core of the Mother.

And so it is, and so it is, and so it is.

HOSPITAL

◑ (Projecting) We are placing _____(Name and Address of Hospital) in an orb with mirrors facing in and mirrors facing out, the Sirius B Council on the outside, Archangels Raphael, Uriel, Gabriel, and Michael at the four cardinal points.

We are placing a containment orb to the right of the main orb with mirrors facing in and mirrors facing out, the Sirius B Council on the outside, Archangels Raphael, Uriel, Gabriel, and Michael at the four cardinal points.

We invoke all the Ascended Masters and Angelic Beings of the Universe to go up as a conduit, through the Galactic Core, Central Sun, Secret Sun, Platinum Sun, into conscious, subconscious, and all altered states of consciousness, and come down into _____ (Name and Address of Hospital).

◐ (Extracting) We are clearing all furniture, fixtures, medical appliances, medical instruments, pharmaceuticals, and extracting all trauma, pain, suffering that had been internalized in _____ (Name and Address of Hospital), all hospital departments, patient rooms, support service operations such as food service prep areas and restaurants, snack bars, and vending machines, security offices, banking ATMs, housekeeping stations, operations offices, maintenance areas, from the manifest to the unmanifest, from particle to wave, transmuting to a neutral energy. Clearing all EMF energy fluctuations from solar flares and geomagnetic storms, cellular transmissions, and all forms of radiation, in matter, dark matter, antimatter, energy, space, time, and all alternate realities, mind control, non-beneficial interdimensional beings, earthbound tricksters, extraterrestrials, artificial intelligence, subliminal messages, hypnosis and posthypnotic suggestions in all forms, parasites, viruses, non-beneficial bacteria, collective-consciousness fear, anxiety, trauma, emotional charges, cords, attachments, implants, hooks, entities, and thought forms, seen or unseen, cloaked or uncloaked, in conscious, subconscious, and all altered states of consciousness, even if they are changing frequencies and dimensions, simultaneously, in matter, dark matter, antimatter, energy, space, time, and all alternate realities. We are moving everything into the containment orb at the count of 10.

1, 2, 3, 4, 5, 6, 7, 8, 9, 10 - Increasing the cohesion to the 987th Fibonacci number.

We are clearing all imprints, echoes, residuals, energetic tattoos associated with what we just cleared, simultaneously, in matter, dark matter, antimatter, energy, space, time, and all alternate realities. We are moving everything into the containment orb at the count of 10.

1, 2, 3, 4, 5, 6, 7, 8, 9, 10 - Increasing the cohesion to the 987th Fibonacci number.

↷ (Projecting) We are sealing the containment orb.

↶ (Extracting) Sending it to the Central Sun.

And so it is, and so it is, and so it is.

ORGAN TRANSPLANTS

◗ (Projecting) We are placing _____(Name of Organ Recipient) and the donated organ on a horizontal podium, inside an orb with mirrors facing in and mirrors facing out, the Sirius B Council on the outside, Archangels Raphael, Uriel, Gabriel, and Michael at the four cardinal points.

We are placing a containment orb to the right of the main orb with mirrors facing in and mirrors facing out, the Sirius B Council on the outside, Archangels Raphael, Uriel, Gabriel, and Michael at the four cardinal points.

We invoke all the Ascended Masters and Angelic Beings of the Universe to go up as a conduit, through the Galactic Core, Central Sun, Secret Sun, Platinum Sun, into conscious, subconscious, and all altered states of consciousness, and come down into _____ (Name of Organ Recipient). We are merging the donated organ with the organ recipient into one energy field.

◖ (Extracting) We are clearing the recipient soul of all energetic imbalances between the donated organ and the organ recipient, from the manifest to the unmanifest, from particle to wave, transmuting to a neutral energy. Clearing all EMF energy fluctuations from solar flares and geomagnetic storms, cellular transmissions, and all forms of radiation, in matter, dark matter, antimatter, energy, space, time, and all alternate realities, mind control, non-beneficial interdimensional beings, earthbound tricksters, extraterrestrials, artificial intelligence, subliminal messages, hypnosis and posthypnotic suggestions in all forms, parasites, viruses, non-beneficial bacteria, collective-consciousness fear, anxiety, trauma, emotional charges, cords, attachments, implants, hooks, entities, and thought forms, seen or unseen, cloaked or uncloaked, in conscious, subconscious, and all altered states of consciousness, even if they are changing frequencies and dimensions between _____(Name of Organ Recipient) and the donated organ, simultaneously, in matter,

dark matter, antimatter, energy, space, time, and all alternate realities. We are moving everything into the containment orb at the count of 10.

1, 2, 3, 4, 5, 6, 7, 8, 9, 10 - Increasing the cohesion to the 987th Fibonacci number.

We are clearing all imprints, echoes, residuals, energetic tattoos associated with what we just cleared, simultaneously, in matter, dark matter, antimatter, energy, space, time, and all alternate realities. We are moving everything into the containment orb at the count of 10.

1, 2, 3, 4, 5, 6, 7, 8, 9, 10 - Increasing the cohesion to the 987th Fibonacci number.

↷ (Projecting) We are sealing the containment orb.

↶ (Extracting) Sending it to the Central Sun.

↷ (Projecting) We invoke all the Ascended Masters and Angelic Beings of the Universe to go up as a conduit, through the Galactic Core, Central Sun, Secret Sun, Platinum Sun, in conscious, subconscious, and all altered states of consciousness, to equalize the donated organ to the same vibration, frequency and dimension at which the organ recipient currently vibrates, and to bind and transmute the donated organ's DNA and genetic coding to the DNA and genetic coding of the recipient.

And so it is, and so it is, and so it is.

PATIENT ROOM

◯ (Projecting) We are placing _____(Patient and Building/ Room Number) in an orb with mirrors facing in and mirrors facing out, the Sirius B Council on the outside, Archangels Raphael, Uriel, Gabriel, and Michael at the four cardinal points.

We are placing a containment orb to the right of the main orb with mirrors facing in and mirrors facing out, the Sirius B Council on the outside, Archangels Raphael, Uriel, Gabriel, and Michael at the four cardinal points.

We invoke all the Ascended Masters and Angelic Beings of the Universe to go up as a conduit, through the Galactic Core, Central Sun, Secret Sun, Platinum Sun, into conscious, subconscious, and all altered states of consciousness, and come down into _____ (Patient and Building/Room Number).

◯ (Extracting) We are clearing _____(Patient and Building/ Room number), all furniture, fixtures, medical appliances, medical instruments, pharmaceuticals, and extracting all trauma, pain, suffering that had been internalized in _____(Patient and Building/Room Number), from the manifest to the unmanifest, from particle to wave, transmuting to a neutral energy. Clearing all EMF energy fluctuations from solar flares and geomagnetic storms, cellular transmissions, and all forms of radiation, in matter, dark matter, antimatter, energy, space, time, and all alternate realities, mind control, non-beneficial interdimensional beings, earthbound tricksters, extraterrestrials, artificial intelligence, subliminal messages, hypnosis and posthypnotic suggestions in all forms, parasites, viruses, non-beneficial bacteria, collective-consciousness fear, anxiety, trauma, emotional charges, cords, attachments, implants, hooks, entities, and thought forms, seen or unseen, cloaked or uncloaked, in conscious, subconscious, and all altered states of consciousness, even if they are changing frequencies and dimensions in _____(Patient and Building/Room Number), simultaneously, in matter, dark matter, antimatter, energy, space, time, and all alternate realities. We are moving everything into the containment orb at the count of 10.

1, 2, 3, 4, 5, 6, 7, 8, 9, 10 - Increasing the cohesion to the 987th Fibonacci number.

We are clearing all imprints, echoes, residuals, energetic tattoos associated with what we just cleared, simultaneously, in matter, dark matter, antimatter, energy, space, time, and all alternate realities. We are moving everything into the containment orb at the count of 10.

1, 2, 3, 4, 5, 6, 7, 8, 9, 10 - Increasing the cohesion to the 987th Fibonacci number.

↻ (Projecting) We are sealing the containment orb.

↺ (Extracting) Sending it to the Central Sun.

And so it is, and so it is, and so it is.

PHANTOM ORGANS

☽ (Projecting) We are placing _____(Phantom Organ) of _____(Name) inside an orb with mirrors facing in and mirrors facing out, the Sirius B Council on the outside, Archangels Raphael, Uriel, Gabriel, and Michael at the four cardinal points.

We are placing a containment orb to the right of the main orb with mirrors facing in and mirrors facing out, the Sirius B Council on the outside, Archangels Raphael, Uriel, Gabriel, and Michael at the four cardinal points.

We invoke all the Ascended Masters and Angelic Beings of the Universe to go up as a conduit, through the Galactic Core, Central Sun, Secret Sun, Platinum Sun, into conscious, subconscious, and all altered states of consciousness, and come down into the _____ (Phantom Organ).

☾ (Extracting) We are clearing all trauma, fear, pain, emotional charges, sense of loss and imbalances from the loss of the _____ (Phantom Organ), from the manifest to the unmanifest, from particle to wave, transmuting to a neutral energy. We are clearing all EMF energy fluctuations from solar flares and geomagnetic storms, cellular transmissions, and all forms of radiation, in matter, dark matter, antimatter, energy, space, time, and all alternate realities, mind control, non-beneficial interdimensional beings, earthbound tricksters, extraterrestrials, artificial intelligence, subliminal messages, hypnosis and posthypnotic suggestions in all forms, parasites, viruses, non-beneficial bacteria, collective-consciousness fear, anxiety, trauma, emotional charges, cords, attachments, implants, hooks, entities, and thought forms, seen or unseen, cloaked or uncloaked, in conscious, subconscious, and all altered states of consciousness, even if they are changing frequencies and dimensions in _____(Name), simultaneously, in matter, dark matter, antimatter, energy, space, time, and all alternate realities. We are moving everything into the containment orb at the count of 10.

1, 2, 3, 4, 5, 6, 7, 8, 9, 10 - Increasing the cohesion to the 987th Fibonacci number.

We are clearing all imprints, echoes, residuals, energetic tattoos associated with what we just cleared, simultaneously, in matter, dark matter, antimatter, energy, space, time, and all alternate realities. We are moving everything into the containment orb at the count of 10.

1, 2, 3, 4, 5, 6, 7, 8, 9, 10 - Increasing the cohesion to the 987th Fibonacci number.

◯ (Projecting) We are sealing the containment orb.

◯ (Extracting) Sending it to the Central Sun.

◯ (Projecting) We invoke all the Ascended Masters and Angelic Beings of the Universe to go up as a conduit, through the Galactic Core, Central Sun, Secret Sun, Platinum Sun, in conscious, subconscious, and all altered states of consciousness, to restore the _____ (Phantom Organ) to full holographic functionality in synchronicity with the other organs of the body.

And so it is, and so it is, and so it is.

PRE-OP SURGERY

◗ (Projecting) We are placing _____(Location of the Operating Room) in an orb with mirrors facing in and mirrors facing out, the Sirius B Council on the outside, Archangels Raphael, Uriel, Gabriel, and Michael at the four cardinal points.

We are placing a containment orb to the right of the main orb, with mirrors facing in and mirrors facing out, the Sirius B Council on the outside, Archangels Raphael, Uriel, Gabriel, and Michael at the four cardinal points.

We invoke all the Ascended Masters and Angelic Beings of the Universe to go up as a conduit, through the Galactic Core, Central Sun, Secret Sun, Platinum Sun, into conscious, subconscious, and all altered states of consciousness, and come down into the _____ (Location of the Operating Room).

◖ (Extracting) We are clearing all furniture, fixtures, medical appliances, medical instruments, pharmaceuticals, and extracting all trauma, pain, suffering, and emotional charges of all kinds that have been internalized in the _____(Location of the Operating Room), from the manifest to the unmanifest, from particle to wave, transmuting to a neutral energy. Clearing all EMF energy fluctuations from solar flares and geomagnetic storms, cellular transmissions, and all forms of radiation, in matter, dark matter, antimatter, energy, space, time, and all alternate realities, mind control, non-beneficial interdimensional beings, earthbound tricksters, extraterrestrials, artificial intelligence, subliminal messages, hypnosis and posthypnotic suggestions in all forms, parasites, viruses, non-beneficial bacteria, collective-consciousness fear, anxiety, trauma, emotional charges, cords, attachments, implants, hooks, entities, and thought forms, seen or unseen, cloaked or uncloaked, in conscious, subconscious, and all altered states of consciousness, even if they are changing frequencies and dimensions, simultaneously, in matter,

dark matter, antimatter, energy, space, time, and all alternate realities. We are moving everything into the containment orb at the count of 10.

1, 2, 3, 4, 5, 6, 7, 8, 9, 10 - Increasing the cohesion to the 987th Fibonacci number.

We are clearing all imprints, echoes, residuals, energetic tattoos associated with what we just cleared, simultaneously, in matter, dark matter, antimatter, energy, space, time, and all alternate realities. We are moving everything into the containment orb at the count of 10.

1, 2, 3, 4, 5, 6, 7, 8, 9, 10 - Increasing the cohesion to the 987th Fibonacci number.

◗ (Projecting) We are sealing the containment orb.

◖ (Extracting) Sending it to the Central Sun.

And so it is, and so it is, and so it is.

PSYCHIC SURGERY

☽ (Projecting) We are placing _____(Surgeon's Name) in an orb with mirrors facing in and mirrors facing out, the Sirius B Council on the outside, Archangels Raphael, Uriel, Gabriel, and Michael at the four cardinal points.

We are placing a containment orb to the right of the main orb with mirrors facing in and mirrors facing out, the Sirius B Council on the outside, Archangels Raphael, Uriel, Gabriel, and Michael at the four cardinal points.

We invoke all the Ascended Masters and Angelic Beings of the Universe to go up as a conduit, through the Galactic Core, Central Sun, Secret Sun, Platinum Sun, into conscious, subconscious, and all altered states of consciousness, and come down into _____ (Surgeon's Name).

☾ (Extracting) We ask for the best possible surgical outcome and to energetically clear _____(Surgeon's Name) of all emotional charges or imbalances which could adversely affect the outcome of the surgery, from the manifest to the unmanifest, from particle to wave, transmuting to a neutral energy. Clearing all EMF energy fluctuations from solar flares and geomagnetic storms, cellular transmissions, and all forms of radiation, in matter, dark matter, antimatter, energy, space, time, and all alternate realities, mind control, non-beneficial interdimensional beings, earthbound trick-sters, extraterrestrials, artificial intelligence, subliminal messages, hypnosis and posthypnotic suggestions in all forms, parasites, viruses, non-beneficial bacteria, collective-consciousness fear, anxiety, trauma, emotional charges, cords, attachments, implants, hooks, entities, and thought forms, seen or unseen, cloaked or uncloaked, in conscious, subconscious, and all altered states of consciousness, even if they are changing frequencies and dimensions, simultane-ously, in matter, dark matter, antimatter, energy, space, time, and all alternate realities. We are moving everything into the containment orb at the of 10.

1, 2, 3, 4, 5, 6, 7, 8, 9, 10 - Increasing the cohesion to the 987th Fibonacci number.

We are clearing all imprints, echoes, residuals, energetic tattoos associated with what we just cleared, simultaneously, in matter, dark matter, antimatter, energy, space, time, and all alternate realities. We are moving everything into the containment orb at the count of 10.

1, 2, 3, 4, 5, 6, 7, 8, 9, 10 - Increasing the cohesion to the 987th Fibonacci number.

⟳ (Projecting) We are sealing the containment orb.

⟲ (Extracting) Sending it to the Central Sun.

⟳ (Projecting) We invoke all the Ascended Masters and Angelic Beings of the Universe to go up as a conduit, through the Galactic Core, Central Sun, Secret Sun, Platinum Sun, into conscious, subconscious, and all altered states of consciousness, and down into _____(Surgeon's Name) eyes, ears, mind, and hands for the best possible outcome for _____(Patient's Name).

And so it is, and so it is, and so it is.

VIRUS, VACCINES, AND BOOSTERS MITIGATION

☌ (Projecting) We are placing _____(Name) in an orb with mirrors facing in and mirrors facing out, the Sirius B Council on the outside, Archangels Raphael, Uriel, Gabriel, and Michael at the four cardinal points.

We are placing a containment orb to the right of the main orb with mirrors facing in and mirror facing out, the Sirius B Council on the outside, Archangels Raphael, Uriel, Gabriel, and Michael at the four cardinal points.

We invoke all the Ascended Masters and Angelic Beings of the Universe to go up as a conduit, through the Galactic Core, Central Sun, Secret Sun, Platinum Sun, into conscious, subconscious, and all altered states of consciousness, and come down into _____ (Name).

☽ (Extracting) We are clearing _____(Name) of fear, anxiety, and trauma from family, friends, acquaintances, neighbors, coworkers, and social media contacts who are aware that _____(Name) has the virus and/or vaccines and boosters. We are internally clearing heavy metals and all toxicity from the virus and/or vaccines and boosters out of all the vital organs and the cellular DNA throughout the body. We are clearing out all residual low-vibrational energy residing in the physical body, from the manifest to the unmanifest, from particle to wave, transmuting to a neutral energy. Clearing all EMF energy fluctuations from solar flares and geomagnetic storms, cellular transmissions, and all forms of radiation, in matter, dark matter, antimatter, energy, space, time, and all alternate realities, mind control, non-beneficial interdimensional beings, earthbound tricksters, extraterrestrials, artificial intelligence, subliminal messages, hypnosis and posthypnotic suggestions in all forms, parasites, viruses, non-beneficial bacteria, collective-consciousness fear, anxiety, trauma, emotional charges, cords, attachments, implants, hooks, entities, and thought forms, seen or unseen, cloaked or uncloaked, in conscious, subconscious, and all altered states of consciousness, even if they are changing frequencies and dimensions, simultaneously, in matter, dark matter, antimatter, energy, space, time, and all alternate realities. We are moving everything into the containment orb at the count of 10.

1, 2, 3, 4, 5, 6, 7, 8, 9, 10 - Increasing the cohesion to the 987th Fibonacci number.

We are clearing all imprints, echoes, residuals, energetic tattoos associated with what we just cleared, simultaneously, in matter, dark matter, antimatter, energy, space, time, and all alternate realities. We are moving everything into the containment orb at the count of 10.

1, 2, 3, 4, 5, 6, 7, 8, 9, 10 - Increasing the cohesion to the 987th Fibonacci number.

↷ (Projecting) We are sealing the containment orb.

↶ (Extracting) Sending it to the Central Sun.

↷ (Projecting) We invoke all the Ascended Masters and Angelic Beings of the Universe to go up to go up as a conduit, through the Galactic Core, Central Sun, Secret Sun, Platinum Sun, into conscious, subconscious, and all altered states of consciousness, and down into _____(Name) holographic higher self at the time of conception in this incarnation and overlay the hologram of the higher self in the physical body, anchoring the holographic higher self into the physical body and fully grounding into the crystal core of the Mother.

And so it is, and so it is, and so it is.

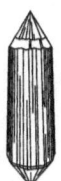

CHAPTER 6

RESETTING PAST MATTERS

CORD CUTTING

☽ (Projecting) We are placing _____(First Person's Name) and _____(Second Person's Name) on a horizontal podium, inside an orb with mirrors facing in and mirrors facing out, the Sirius B Council on the outside, Archangels Raphael, Uriel, Gabriel, and Michael at the four cardinal points.

We are placing a containment orb to the right of the main orb with mirrors facing in and mirrors facing out, the Sirius B Council on the outside, Archangels Raphael, Uriel, Gabriel, and Michael at the four cardinal points.

We invoke all the Ascended Masters and Angelic Beings of the Universe to go up as a conduit, through the Galactic Core, Central Sun, Secret Sun, Platinum Sun, into conscious, subconscious, and all altered states of consciousness, and come down into _____ (First Person's Name) and _____(Second Person's Name)

☾ (Extracting) We are cutting all cords between _____(First Person's Name) and _____(Second Person's Name) and all emotional charges, from the manifest to the unmanifest, from particle to wave, transmuting to a neutral energy. Clearing all EMF energy fluctuations from solar flares and geomagnetic storms, cellular transmissions, and all forms of radiation, in matter, dark matter, antimatter, energy, space, time, and all alternate realities, mind control, non-beneficial interdimensional beings, earthbound tricksters, extraterrestrials, artificial intelligence, subliminal messages, hypnosis and posthypnotic suggestions in all forms, parasites, viruses, non-beneficial bacteria, collective-consciousness fear, anxiety, trauma, emotional charges, cords, attachments, implants, hooks, entities, and thought forms, seen or unseen, cloaked or uncloaked, in conscious, subconscious, and all altered states of consciousness, even if they are changing frequencies and dimensions, simultaneously, in matter, dark matter, antimatter, energy, space, time, and all alternate

realities. We are moving everything into the containment orb at the count of 10.

1, 2, 3, 4, 5, 6, 7, 8, 9, 10 - Increasing the cohesion to the 987th Fibonacci number.

We are clearing all imprints, echoes, residuals, energetic tattoos associated with what we just cleared, simultaneously, in matter, dark matter, antimatter, energy, space, time, and all alternate realities. We are moving everything into the containment orb at the count of 10.

1, 2, 3, 4, 5, 6, 7, 8, 9, 10 - Increasing the cohesion to the 987th Fibonacci number.

↷ (Projecting) We are sealing the containment orb.

↶ (Extracting) Sending it to the Central Sun.

And so it is, and so it is, and so it is.

EXPOSING/UNMASKING

◑ (Projecting) We are placing _____(Name of Person, Object or Location) in an orb with mirrors facing in and mirrors facing out, the Sirius B Council on the outside, Archangels Raphael, Uriel, Gabriel, and Michael at the four cardinal points.

We invoke all the Ascended Masters and Angelic beings of the Universe to go up as a conduit, through the Galactic Core, Central Sun, Secret Sun, Platinum Sun, into conscious, subconscious, and all altered states of consciousness, and bring 987 trillion Broadway spotlights, shining them over, under and around _____(Name of Person, Object or Location), lighting and uncloaking and unmasking all aspects of what _____(Name of Person, Object or Location) is doing and everything going on that has been hidden, camouflaged, or kept secret, so it will be common knowledge and transparent.

◐ (Extracting) We invoke the Ascended Masters and Angelic Beings to go up as a conduit, through the Galactic Core, Central Sun, Secret Sun, Platinum Sun, in conscious, subconscious, and all altered states of consciousness, and down into _____(Name of Person, Object or Location) to totally uncloak and unmask.

◑ (Projecting) Bringing to the light everything going on so it can be seen clearly.

And so it is, and so it is, and so it is.

GENETIC LINEAGE AND ANCESTRAL DNA

☽ (Projecting) We are placing _____(Name) in an orb with mirrors facing in and mirrors facing out; the Sirius B Council on the outside, Archangels Raphael, Uriel, Gabriel, and Michael at the four cardinal points.

We are placing a containment orb to the right of the main orb with mirrors facing in and mirrors facing out, the Sirius B Council on the outside, Archangels Raphael, Uriel, Gabriel, and Michael at the four cardinal points.

We invoke all the Ascended Masters and Angelic Beings of the Universe to go up as a conduit, through the Galactic Core, Central Sun, Secret Sun, Platinum Sun, into conscious, subconscious, and all altered states of consciousness, and come down into the maternal and paternal lineages from the beginning of time, and come down into _____(Name).

☾ (Extracting) We are clearing _____(Name) of the emotional charges of all ancestors of both the maternal and paternal lineages from the beginning of time, through all generations, past lives, this life, concurrent lives, alternative lives, parallel lives, and future lives, and clearing any distortion coming through into this life. We are disconnecting and removing all emotional trauma from past lives, this life, concurrent lives, alternative lives, parallel lives, and future lives, as well as all emotional trauma from ancestors passed down in the genetic coding of the cellular DNA of _____(Name), from the manifest to the unmanifest, from particle to wave, transmuting to a neutral energy, seen or unseen, cloaked or uncloaked, in conscious, subconscious, and all altered states of consciousness, even if they are changing frequencies and dimensions, simultaneously, in matter, dark matter, antimatter, energy, space, time, and all alternate

realities. We are moving everything into the containment orb at the count of 10.

   1, 2, 3, 4, 5, 6, 7, 8, 9, 10 - Increasing the cohesion to the 987th Fibonacci number.

   We are clearing all imprints, echoes, residuals, energetic tattoos associated with what we just cleared, simultaneously, in matter, dark matter, antimatter, energy, space, time, and all alternate realities. We are moving everything into the containment orb at the count of 10.

   1, 2, 3, 4, 5, 6, 7, 8, 9, 10 - Increasing the cohesion to the 987th Fibonacci number.

↷ (Projecting) We are sealing the containment orb.

↶ (Extracting) Sending it to the Central Sun.

   And so it is, and so it is, and so it is.

PAST LIVES

◖ (Projecting) We are placing _____(Name) in an orb with mirrors facing in and mirrors facing out, the Sirius B Council on the outside, Archangels Raphael, Uriel, Gabriel, and Michael at the four cardinal points.

We are placing a containment orb to the right of the main orb with mirrors facing in and mirrors facing out, the Sirius B Council on the outside, Archangels Raphael, Uriel, Gabriel, and Michael at the four cardinal points.

We invoke all the Ascended Masters and Angelic Beings of the Universe to go up as a conduit, through the Galactic Core, Central Sun, Secret Sun, Platinum Sun, into conscious, subconscious, and all altered states of consciousness, and come down into _____ (Name).

◖ (Extracting) We are clearing _____(Name) of all past-life emotional charges, cords, attachments, implants, hooks, entities, and thought forms that have imprinted trauma from past lives into this life, from the manifest to the unmanifest, from particle to wave, transmuting to a neutral energy, seen or unseen, cloaked or uncloaked, even if they are changing frequencies and dimensions, simultaneously, in matter, dark matter, antimatter, energy, space, time, and all alternate realities. We are moving everything into the containment orb at the count of 10.

1, 2, 3, 4, 5, 6, 7, 8, 9, 10 - Increasing the cohesion to the 987th Fibonacci number.

We are clearing all imprints, echoes, residuals, energetic tattoos associated with what we just cleared, simultaneously, in matter, dark matter, antimatter, energy, space, time, and all alternate realities. We are moving everything into the containment orb at the count of 10.

1, 2, 3, 4, 5, 6, 7, 8, 9, 10 - Increasing the cohesion to the 987th Fibonacci me) number.

↷ (Projecting) We are sealing the containment orb.

↶ (Extracting) Sending it to the Central Sun.

↷ (Projecting) We invoke all the Ascended Masters and Angelic Beings of the Universe to go up as a conduit, through the Galactic Core, Central Sun, Secret Sun, Platinum Sun, into conscious, subconscious, and all altered states of consciousness, and to stream glittering, shimmering Galactic Light into the cellular DNA of _____ (Name), raising the vibration and frequency to the highest vibration and frequency _____(Name) can accept, anchoring the holographic higher self into the physical body and fully grounding into the crystal core of the Mother.

And so it is, and so it is, and so it is.

RELATIONSHIP RESETS

↻ (Projecting) We are placing _____(First Person's Name) on the right and _____(Second Person's Name) on the left on a horizontal podium in an orb with mirrors facing in and mirrors facing out, the Sirius B Council on the outside, Archangels Raphael, Uriel, Gabriel, and Michael at the four cardinal points.

We are placing a containment orb to the right of the main orb with mirrors facing in and mirrors facing out, the Sirius B Council on the outside, Archangels Raphael, Uriel, Gabriel, and Michael at the four cardinal points.

We invoke all the Ascended Masters and Angelic Beings of the Universe to go up as a conduit, through the Galactic Core, Central Sun, Secret Sun, Platinum Sun, into conscious, subconscious, and all altered states of consciousness, and come down into _____ (First Person's Name) and into _____(Second Person's Name).

↻ (Extracting) We are clearing _____(First Person's Name) and _____(Second Person's Name) of any conflicts, emotional charges and misunderstandings, from the manifest to the unmanifest, from particle to wave, transmuting to a neutral energy. Clearing all EMF energy fluctuations from solar flares and geomagnetic storms, cellular transmissions, and all forms of radiation, in matter, dark matter, antimatter, energy, space, time, and all alternate realities, mind control, non-beneficial interdimensional beings, earthbound tricksters, extraterrestrials, artificial intelligence, subliminal messages, hypnosis and posthypnotic suggestions in all forms, parasites, viruses, non-beneficial bacteria, collective-consciousness fear, anxiety, trauma, emotional charges, cords, attachments, implants, hooks, entities, and thought forms, seen or unseen, cloaked or uncloaked, in conscious, subconscious, and all altered states of consciousness, even if they are changing frequencies and dimensions, simultaneously, in matter, dark matter, antimatter, energy, space, time, and all alternate realities. We are moving everything into the containment orb at the count of 10.

1, 2, 3, 4, 5, 6, 7, 8, 9, 10 - Increasing the cohesion to the 987th Fibonacci number.

We are clearing all imprints, echoes, residuals, energetic tattoos associated with what we just cleared, simultaneously, in matter, dark matter, antimatter, energy, space, time, and all alternate realities. We are moving everything into the containment orb at the count of 10.

1, 2, 3, 4, 5, 6, 7, 8, 9, 10 - Increasing the cohesion to the 987th Fibonacci number.

◠ (Projecting) We are sealing the containment orb.

◠ (Extracting) Sending it to the Central Sun.

◠ (Projecting) We make a horizontal infinity symbol, with galactic light code, looping one side around _____(First Person's Name) and the other loop around _____(Second Person's Name), and then we merge both people into one energy field.

And so it is, and so it is, and so it is.

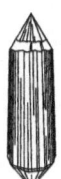

CHAPTER 7

RELEASING TRAUMAS

ABUSE AND TRAUMA

◗ (Projecting) We are placing _____(Name) in an orb with mirrors facing in and mirrors facing out, the Sirius B Council on the outside, Archangels Raphael, Uriel, Gabriel, and Michael at the four cardinal points.

We are placing a containment orb to the right of the main orb with mirrors facing in and mirrors facing out, the Sirius B Council on the outside, Archangels Raphael, Uriel, Gabriel, and Michael at the four cardinal points.

We invoke all the Ascended Masters and Angelic Beings of the Universe to go up as a conduit, through the Galactic Core, Central Sun, Secret Sun, Platinum Sun into conscious, subconscious, and all altered states of consciousness and come down into _____ (Name).

◖ (Extracting) We are clearing _____(Name) of the emotional charges in their cellular DNA and of all other forms of abuse in matter, dark matter, antimatter, energy, space, time, and all alternate realities, from the manifest to the unmanifest, from particle to wave, transmuting to a neutral energy. Clearing all EMF energy fluctuations from solar flares and geomagnetic storms, cellular transmissions, and all forms of radiation, in matter, dark matter, antimatter, energy, space, time, and all alternate realities, mind control, non-beneficial interdimensional beings, earthbound tricksters, extraterrestrials, artificial intelligence, subliminal messages, hypnosis and posthypnotic suggestions in all forms, collective consciousness fear, anxiety, trauma, emotional charges, cords, attachments, implants, hooks, entities, and thought forms, seen or unseen, cloaked or uncloaked, in conscious, subconscious, and all altered states of consciousness, even if they are changing frequencies and dimensions, simultaneously, in matter, dark matter, antimatter, energy, space, time, and all alternate realities. We are moving everything into the containment orb at the count of 10.

1, 2, 3, 4, 5, 6, 7, 8, 9, 10 - Increasing the cohesion to the 987th Fibonacci number.

We are clearing all imprints, echoes, residuals, energetic tattoos associated with what we just cleared, simultaneously, in matter, dark matter, antimatter, energy, space, time, and all alternate realities. We are moving everything into the containment orb at the count of 10.

1, 2, 3, 4, 5, 6, 7, 8, 9, 10 - Increasing the cohesion to the 987th Fibonacci number.

↷ (Projecting) We are sealing the containment orb.

↶ (Extracting) Sending it to the Central Sun.

↷ (Projecting) We invoke all the Ascended Masters and Angelic Beings of the Universe to go up as a conduit, through the Galactic Core, Central Sun, Secret Sun, Platinum Sun, into conscious, subconscious, and all altered states of consciousness, with Ruby Red light and eucalyptus saplings, and go down into _____(Name). We restore _____(Name) to the emotionally zero-pointed neutral state (he/she/they) were in at the time of conception in this incarnation and to the emotional health _____(Name) had at the moment of conception, anchoring the holographic higher self into the physical body and fully grounding into the crystal core of the Mother.

And so it is, and so it is, and so it is.

ADDICTION

↻ (Projecting) We are placing _____(Name) in an orb with mirrors facing in and mirrors facing out, the Sirius B Council on the outside, Archangels Raphael, Uriel, Gabriel, and Michael at the four cardinal points.

We are placing a containment orb to the right of the main orb with mirrors facing in and mirrors facing out, the Sirius B Council on the outside, Archangels Raphael, Uriel, Gabriel, and Michael at the four cardinal points.

We invoke all the Ascended Masters and Angelic Beings of the universe, to go up as a conduit, through the Galactic Core, Central Sun, Secret Sun, Platinum Sun, into conscious, subconscious, and all altered states of consciousness, and come down into _____(Name).

↻ (Extracting) We are clearing _____(Name) of the entities and demons from their addiction, empathic and emotional trauma, blame, the story, humiliation, fear, and anxiety associated with the events which they do not want to remember out of their cellular DNA, from the manifest to the unmanifest, from particle to wave, transmuting to a neutral energy. Clearing all EMF energy fluctuations from solar flares and geomagnetic storms, cellular transmissions, and all forms of radiation, in matter, dark matter, antimatter, energy, space, time, and all alternate realities, mind control, non-beneficial interdimensional beings, earthbound tricksters, extraterrestrials, artificial intelligence, subliminal messages, hypnosis and posthypnotic suggestions in all forms, collective-consciousness fear, anxiety, trauma, emotional charges, cords, attachments, implants, hooks, entities, and thought forms, seen or unseen, cloaked or uncloaked, in conscious, subconscious, and all altered states of consciousness, even if they are changing frequencies and dimensions, simultaneously, in matter, dark matter, antimatter, energy, space, time, and all alternate

realities. We are moving everything into the containment orb at the count of 10.

1, 2, 3, 4, 5, 6, 7, 8, 9, 10 - Increasing the cohesion to the 987th Fibonacci number.

We are clearing all imprints, echoes, residuals, energetic tattoos associated with what we just cleared, in matter, dark matter, antimatter, energy, space, time, and all alternate realities. We are moving everything into the containment orb at the count of 10.

1, 2, 3, 4, 5, 6, 7, 8, 9, 10 - Increasing the cohesion to the 987th Fibonacci number.

(Projecting) We are sealing the containment orb.

(Extracting) Sending it to the Central Sun.

(Projecting) We invoke the Ascended Masters and Angelic Beings to go up as a conduit, through the Galactic Core, Central Sun, Secret Sun, Platinum Sun, into conscious, subconscious, and all altered states of consciousness, taking Ruby Red light and eucalyptus saplings, and go down into _____(Name) and anchor the holographic higher self into the physical body, assuming the emotional health (he/she/they) had before they experienced the addiction, restoring _____(Name) to a neutral energy without the addictive emotional charges, as they were at the age of conception in this incarnation, anchoring the holographic higher self into the physical body and fully grounding into the crystal core of the Mother.

And so it is, and so it is, and so it is.

BLOCKED CHAKRAS

◖ (Projecting) We are placing _____(Name) in an orb with mirror facing in and mirrors facing out, the Sirius B Council on the outside, and Archangels Raphael, Uriel, Gabriel, and Michael at the four cardinal points.

We are placing a containment orb to the right of the main orb with mirrors facing in and mirrors facing out, the Sirius B Council on the outside, Archangels Raphael, Uriel, Gabriel, and Michael at the four cardinal points.

We invoke all the Ascended Masters and Angelic Beings of the Universe to go up as a conduit, through the Galactic Core, Central Sun, Secret Sun, Platinum Sun, into conscious, subconscious, and all altered states of consciousness and come down into the Crown, Third Eye, Throat, Heart, Solar Plexus, Sacral, and Root Chakras individually and come down into _____(Name).

◖ (Extracting) We are clearing _____(Name) and all of the blocked chakras, from the manifest to the unmanifest, from particle to wave, transmuting to a neutral energy. Clearing all EMF energy fluctuations from solar flares and geomagnetic storms, cellular transmissions, and all forms of radiation, in matter, dark matter, antimatter, energy, space, time, and all alternate realities, mind control, non-beneficial interdimensional beings, earthbound tricksters, extraterrestrials, artificial intelligence, subliminal messages, hypnosis and posthypnotic suggestions in all forms, collective-consciousness fear, anxiety, trauma, emotional charges, cords, attachments, implants, hooks, entities, and thought forms, seen or unseen, cloaked or uncloaked, in conscious, subconscious, and all altered states of consciousness, even if they are changing frequencies and dimensions, simultaneously, in matter, dark matter, antimatter, energy, space, time, and all alternate realities. We are moving everything into the containment orb at the count of 10.

1, 2, 3, 4, 5, 6, 7, 8, 9, 10 - Increasing the cohesion to the 987th Fibonacci number.

We are clearing all imprints, echoes, residuals, energetic tattoos associated with what we just cleared, simultaneously, in matter, dark matter, antimatter, energy, space, time, and all alternate realities. We are moving everything into the containment orb at the count of 10.

1, 2, 3, 4, 5, 6, 7, 8, 9, 10 - Increasing the cohesion to the 987th Fibonacci number.

◯ (Projecting) We are sealing the containment orb.

◯ (Extracting) Sending it to the Central Sun.

◯ (Projecting) We invoke the Ascended Masters and Angelic Beings to go up as a conduit, through the Galactic Core, Central Sun, Secret Sun, Platinum Sun, into conscious, subconscious, and all altered states of consciousness, taking Ruby Red light and eucalyptus saplings, and go down into _____(Name) and anchor the holographic higher self into the physical body, assuming the emotional health (he/she/they) had before they experienced the blocked chakras, restoring _____(Name) to a neutral energy without the blocked emotional charges, as they were at the age of conception in this incarnation, anchoring the holographic higher self into the physical body and fully grounding into the crystal core of the Mother.

And so it is, and so it is, and so it is.

EMOTIONAL CHARGES

◯ (Projecting) We are placing _____(Name) in an orb with mirrors facing in and mirrors facing out, the Sirius B Council on the outside, Archangels Raphael, Uriel, Gabriel, and Michael at the four cardinal points.

We are placing a containment orb to the right of the main orb with mirrors facing in and mirrors facing out, the Sirius B Council on the outside, Archangels Raphael, Uriel, Gabriel, and Michael at the four cardinal points.

We invoke all the Ascended Masters and Angelic Beings of the Universe to go up as a conduit, through the Galactic Core, Central Sun, Secret Sun, Platinum Sun, into conscious, subconscious, and all altered states of consciousness, and the holographic higher self of _____(Name) at the time of conception in this incarnation, and go down into _____(Name).

◯ (Extracting) We are clearing _____(Name) of all emotional charges, from the manifest to the unmanifest, from particle to wave, transmuting to a neutral energy. Clearing all EMF energy fluctuations from solar flares and geomagnetic storms, cellular transmissions, and all forms of radiation, in matter, dark matter, antimatter, energy, space, time, and all alternate realities, mind control, non-beneficial interdimensional beings, earthbound tricksters, extraterrestrials, artificial intelligence, subliminal messages, hypnosis and posthyp-notic suggestions in all forms, collective-consciousness fear, anxiety, trauma, emotional charges, cords, attachments, implants, hooks, entities, and thought forms, seen or unseen, cloaked or uncloaked, in conscious, subconscious, and all altered states of consciousness, even if they are changing frequencies and dimensions, simultaneously, in matter, dark matter, antimatter, energy, space, time, and all alternate realities. We are moving everything into the containment orb at the count of 10.

1, 2, 3, 4, 5, 6, 7, 8, 9, 10 - Increasing the cohesion to the 987th Fibonacci number.

We are clearing all imprints, echoes, residuals, energetic tattoos associated with what we just cleared, simultaneously, in matter, dark matter, antimatter, energy, space, time, and all alternate realities. We are moving everything into the containment orb at the count of 10.

1, 2, 3, 4, 5, 6, 7, 8, 9, 10 - Increasing the cohesion to the 987th Fibonacci number.

◯ (Projecting) We are sealing the containment orb.

◯ (Extracting) Sending it to the Central Sun.

◯ (Projecting) We invoke all the Ascended Masters and Angelic Beings of the Universe to go up as a conduit, through the Galactic Core, Central Sun, Secret Sun, Platinum Sun, in conscious, subconscious, and all altered states of consciousness, with Ruby Red light and eucalyptus saplings, to go down into _____(Name). We restore _____(Name) to the emotionally zero-pointed neutral state (he/she/they) were in at the time of conception in this incarnation and to the emotional health _____(Name) had at the moment of conception, anchoring the holographic higher self into the physical body and fully grounding into the crystal core of the Mother.

And so it is, and so it is, and so it is.

FEAR AND CHRONIC PAIN

◑ (Projecting) We are placing _____(Name) in an orb with mirrors facing in and mirrors facing out, the Sirius B Council on the outside, Archangels Raphael, Uriel, Gabriel, and Michael at the four cardinal points.

We are placing a containment orb to the right of the main orb with mirrors facing in and mirrors facing out, the Sirius B Council on the outside, Archangels Raphael, Uriel, Gabriel, and Michael at the four cardinal points.

We invoke all the Ascended Masters and Angelic Beings of the Universe to go up as a conduit, through the Galactic Core, Central Sun, Secret Sun, Platinum Sun and the holographic higher self of _____(Name) at the age of conception in this incarnation and to go down into conscious, subconscious, and all altered states of consciousness and overlay the holographic imprint of the higher self into the physical body and, with Ruby Red light and eucalyptus saplings, go into _____(Name) and anchor the holographic imprint of the higher self into the physical body and ground _____(Name) into the crystal core of the Mother.

◐ (Extracting) We are clearing _____(Name) of all fear and chronic pain, from the manifest to the unmanifest, from particle to wave, transmuting to a neutral energy. Clearing all EMF energy fluctuations from solar flares and geomagnetic storms, cellular transmissions, and all forms of radiation, in matter, dark matter, antimatter, energy, space, time, and all alternate realities, mind control, non-beneficial interdimensional beings, earthbound tricksters, extraterrestrials, artificial intelligence, subliminal messages, hypnosis and posthypnotic suggestions in all forms, collective-consciousness fear, anxiety, trauma, emotional charges, cords, attachments, implants, hooks, entities, and thought forms, seen or unseen, cloaked or uncloaked, in conscious, subconscious, and all altered states of consciousness, even if it is changing frequencies and dimensions, simultaneously, in matter, dark matter, antimatter, energy, space, time, and all alternate realities. We are moving everything into the containment orb at the count of 10.

1, 2, 3, 4, 5, 6, 7, 8, 9, 10 - Increasing the cohesion to the 987th Fibonacci number.

We are clearing all imprints, echoes, residuals, energetic tattoos associated with what we just cleared, simultaneously, in matter, dark matter, antimatter, energy, space, time, and all alternate realities. We are moving everything into the containment orb at the count of 10.

1, 2, 3, 4, 5, 6, 7, 8, 9, 10 - Increasing the cohesion to the 987th Fibonacci number.

☌ (Projecting) We are sealing the containment orb.

☾ (Extracting) Sending it to the Central Sun.

☌ (Projecting) We invoke the Ascended Masters and Angelic Beings to go up as a conduit, through the Galactic Core, Central Sun, Secret Sun, Platinum Sun, into conscious, subconscious, and all altered states of consciousness, taking Ruby Red light and eucalyptus saplings, and go down into _____(Name) and anchor the holographic higher self into the physical body, assuming the emotional health (he/she/they) had before they experienced the fear and trauma, restoring _____(Name) to a neutral energy without the fear, trauma and emotional charges emotional charges, as they were at the age of conception in this incarnation, anchoring the holographic higher self into the physical body and fully grounding into the crystal core of the Mother.

And so it is, And so it is, And so it is.

SEXUAL ABUSE TRAUMA

☽ (Projecting) We are placing _____(Name) in an orb with mirrors facing in and mirrors facing out, the Sirius B Council on the outside, Archangels Raphael, Uriel, Gabriel, and Michael at the four cardinal points.

We are placing a containment orb to the right of the main orb with mirrors facing in and mirrors facing out, the Sirius B Council on the outside, Archangels Raphael, Uriel, Gabriel, and Michael at the four cardinal points.

We invoke all the Ascended Masters and Angelic Beings of the Universe to go up as a conduit, through the Galactic Core, Central Sun, Secret Sun, Platinum Sun, into conscious, subconscious, and all altered states of consciousness, and the holographic higher self of _____(Name) at the time of conception in this incarnation and anchor the holographic higher self in the physical body.

☾ (Extracting) We are clearing _____(Name) of the sexual abuse, internalized trauma in the cellular DNA of the sacral chakra and all the associated emotional charges, from the manifest to the unmanifest, from particle to wave, transmuting to a neutral energy. Clearing all EMF energy fluctuations from solar flares and geomagnetic storms, cellular transmissions, and all forms of radiation, in matter, dark matter, antimatter, energy, space, time, and all alternate realities, mind control, non-beneficial interdimensional beings, earthbound tricksters, extraterrestrials, artificial intelligence, subliminal messages, hypnosis and posthypnotic suggestions in all forms, collective-consciousness fear, anxiety, trauma, emotional charges, cords, attachments, implants, hooks, entities, and thought forms, seen or unseen, cloaked or uncloaked, in conscious, subconscious, and all altered states of consciousness, even if they are changing frequencies and dimensions, simultaneously, in matter, dark matter, antimatter, energy, space, time, and all alternate realities. We are moving everything into the containment orb at the count of 10.

1, 2, 3, 4, 5, 6, 7, 8, 9, 10 - Increasing the cohesion to the 987th Fibonacci number.

We are clearing all imprints, echoes, residuals, energetic tattoos associated with what we just cleared, simultaneously, in matter, dark matter, antimatter, energy, space, time, and all alternate realities. We are moving everything into the containment orb at the count of 10.

1, 2, 3, 4, 5, 6, 7, 8, 9, 10 - Increasing the cohesion to the 987th Fibonacci number.

◗ (Projecting) We are sealing the containment orb.

◖ (Extracting) Sending it to the Central Sun.

◗ (Projecting) We invoke the Ascended Masters and Angelic Beings to go up as a conduit, through the Galactic Core, Central Sun, Secret Sun, Platinum Sun, into conscious, subconscious, and all altered states of consciousness, taking Ruby Red light and eucalyptus saplings, and go down into _____(Name) and anchor the holographic higher self into the physical body, assuming the emotional health (he/she/they) had before they experienced the sexual abuse, restoring _____(Name) to a neutral energy without the sexual abuse and emotional charges, as they were at the age of conception in this incarnation, anchoring the holographic higher self into the physical body and fully grounding into the crystal core of the Mother.

And so it is, and so it is, and so it is.

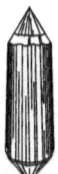

CHAPTER 8
TRANSPORTATION

AIRCRAFT

↻ (Projecting) We are placing __________(Airline & Flight Number) in an orb with mirrors facing in and mirrors facing out, the Sirius B Council on the outside, Archangels Raphael, Uriel, Gabriel, and Michael at the four cardinal points.

We are placing a containment orb to the right of the main orb with mirrors facing in and mirrors facing out, the Sirius B Council on the outside, Archangels Raphael, Uriel, Gabriel, and Michael at the four cardinal points.

We invoke all the Ascended Masters and Angelic Beings of the Universe to go up as a conduit, through the Galactic Core, Central Sun, Secret Sun, Platinum Sun, in conscious, subconscious, and all altered states of consciousness, and then to go down into the __________(Airline & Flight Number).

↺ (Extracting) We are clearing __________(Airline & Flight Number), all onboard passengers, the flight deck captain, the first officer and relief officers, the purser, the lead flight attendant, all other flight attendants and translators, service and transported animals, overhead bins, seats, tray tables, entertainment systems, storage closets, lavatories, galleys, food and beverage carts and equipment, furniture fixtures, and all other personal property, the flight deck, the flight attendants' rest facilities, and the cargo hold on __________ (Airline & Flight Number), from the manifest to the unmanifest, from particle to wave, transmuting to a neutral energy. Clearing all EMF energy fluctuations from solar flares and geomagnetic storms, high speed cellular radiation, cellular transmissions, and all forms of radiation, in matter, dark matter, antimatter, energy, space, time, and all alternate realities, mind control, non-beneficial interdimensional beings, earthbound tricksters, extraterrestrials, artificial intelligence, subliminal messages, hypnosis, post hypnotic suggestions in all forms, collective-consciousness fear, anxiety, trauma, emotional charges, cords, attachments, implants, hooks, entities, and thought forms, seen or unseen, cloaked or uncloaked, in conscious, subconscious, and all altered states of consciousness, even if they are changing frequencies and dimensions, simultaneously, in matter, dark matter, antimatter, energy, space, time, and all alternate realities. We are moving everything into the containment orb at the count of 10.

1, 2, 3, 4, 5, 6, 7, 8, 9, 10 - Increasing the cohesion to the 987th Fibonacci number.

We are clearing all imprints, echoes, residuals, energetic tattoos associated with what we just cleared, simultaneously, in matter, dark matter, antimatter, energy, space, time, and all alternate realities. We are moving everything into the containment orb at the count of 10.

1, 2, 3, 4, 5, 6, 7, 8, 9, 10 - Increasing the cohesion to the 987th Fibonacci number.

◯ (Projecting) We are sealing the containment orb.

◯ (Extracting) Sending it to the Central Sun.

◯ (Projecting) We invoke all the Angelic Beings of the Universe to go up as a conduit the Galactic Core, Central Sun, Secret Sun, Platinum Sun, in conscious, subconscious, and all altered states of consciousness, to place a 100-mile orb around the plane from the time it's airborne to the time it lands to prevent turbulence, porpoising, and inclement weather.

And so it is, and so it is, and so it is.

BUS TOUR

◔ (Projecting) We are placing the tour bus in an orb with mirrors facing in and mirrors facing out, the Sirius B Council on the outside, Archangels Raphael, Uriel, Gabriel, and Michael at the four cardinal points.

We are placing a containment orb to the right of the main orb with mirrors facing in and mirrors facing out, the Sirius B Council on the outside, Archangels Raphael, Uriel, Gabriel, and Michael at the four cardinal points.

We invoke all the Ascended Masters and Angelic Beings of the Universe to go up as a conduit, through the Galactic Core, Central Sun, Secret Sun, Platinum Sun, in conscious, subconscious, and all altered states of consciousness, and then to go down into the tour bus.

◔ (Extracting) We are clearing the tour bus, consisting of the tour bus driver, the passenger(s), tour guide(s), service animals traveling, the passenger compartments, overhead bins, carry-on baggage, seating, entertainment systems, individual seat controls, carpets, lavatory(s), and all other furniture fixtures, as well as the lower baggage storage compartments, from the manifest to the unmanifest, from particle to wave, transmuting to a neutral energy. Clearing all EMF energy fluctuations from solar flares and geomagnetic storms, cellular transmissions, and all forms of radiation, in matter, dark matter, antimatter, energy, space, time, and all alternate realities, mind control, non-beneficial interdimensional beings, earthbound tricksters, extraterrestrials, artificial intelligence, subliminal messages, hypnosis and posthypnotic suggestions in all forms, collective-consciousness fear, anxiety, trauma, emotional charges, cords, attachments, implants, hooks, entities, and thought forms, seen or unseen, cloaked or uncloaked, in conscious, subconscious, and all altered states of consciousness, even if they are changing frequencies and dimensions, simultaneously, in matter, dark matter, antimatter,

energy, space, time, and all alternate realities. We are moving everything into the containment orb at the count of 10.

1, 2, 3, 4, 5, 6, 7, 8, 9, 10 - Increasing the cohesion to the 987th Fibonacci number.

We are clearing all imprints, echoes, residuals, energetic tattoos associated with what we just cleared, simultaneously, in matter, dark matter, antimatter, energy, space, time, and all alternate realities. We are moving everything into the containment orb at the count of 10.

1, 2, 3, 4, 5, 6, 7, 8, 9, 10 - Increasing the cohesion to the 987th Fibonacci number.

☽ (Projecting) We are sealing the containment orb.

☾ (Extracting) Sending it to the Central Sun.

And so it is, and so it is, and so it is.

CARRY-ON AND CHECKED BAGGAGE

◗ (Projecting) We are placing the baggage being transported by
_____(Name) in an orb with mirrors facing in and mirrors
facing out, the Sirius B Council on the outside, Archangels Raphael,
Uriel, Gabriel, and Michael at the four cardinal points.

We are placing a containment orb to the right of the main orb
with mirrors facing in and mirrors facing out, the Sirius B Council
on the outside, Archangels Raphael, Uriel, Gabriel, and Michael at
the four cardinal points.

We invoke all the Ascended Masters and Angelic Beings of the
Universe to go up as a conduit, through the Galactic Core, Central
Sun, Secret Sun, Platinum Sun, in conscious, subconscious, and all
altered states of consciousness, and then to go down into the baggage.

◖ (Extracting) We are clearing all carry-on and checked baggage
being transported by _____(Name), from the manifest to the
unmanifest, from particle to wave, transmuting to a neutral energy.
Clearing all EMF energy fluctuations from solar flares and geomagnetic storms, cellular transmissions, and all forms of radiation, in
matter, dark matter, antimatter, energy, space, time, and all alternate
realities, mind control, non-beneficial interdimensional beings, earthbound tricksters, extraterrestrials, artificial intelligence, subliminal
messages, hypnosis and posthypnotic suggestions in all forms, collective-consciousness fear, anxiety, trauma, emotional charges, cords,
attachments, implants, hooks, entities, and thought forms, seen or
unseen, cloaked or uncloaked, in conscious, subconscious, and all
altered states of consciousness, even if they are changing frequencies
and dimensions, simultaneously, in matter, dark matter, antimatter,
energy, space, time, and all alternate realities. We are moving everything into the containment orb at the count of 10.

1, 2, 3, 4, 5, 6, 7, 8, 9, 10 - Increasing the cohesion to the 987th Fibonacci number.

We are clearing all imprints, echoes, residuals, energetic tattoos associated with what we just cleared, simultaneously, in matter, dark matter, antimatter, energy, space, time, and all alternate realities. We are moving everything into the containment orb at the count of 10.

1, 2, 3, 4, 5, 6, 7, 8, 9, 10 - Increasing the cohesion to the 987th Fibonacci number.

↷ (Projecting) We are sealing the containment orb.

↶ (Extracting) Sending it to the Central Sun.

And so it is, and so it is, and so it is.

CRUISE SHIP

◗ (Projecting) We are placing _____(Cruise Name) in an orb with mirrors facing in and mirrors facing out, the Sirius B Council on the outside, Archangels Raphael, Uriel, Gabriel, and Michael at the four cardinal points.

We are placing a containment orb to the right of the main orb with mirrors facing in and mirrors facing out, the Sirius B Council on the outside, Archangels Raphael, Uriel, Gabriel, and Michael at the four cardinal points.

We invoke all the Ascended Masters and Angelic Beings of the Universe to go up as a conduit, through the Galactic Core, Central Sun, Secret Sun, Platinum Sun, in conscious, subconscious, and all altered states of consciousness, and then to go down into the _____(Cruise Name).

◖ (Extracting) We are clearing _____(Cruise Name), all onboard passengers, cruise officers, crew members and animals on _____(Cruise Name), as well as the passenger and officer/crew rooms, suites and all onboard facilities, lifeboats, swimming pools, restaurants, lounges, casinos, shopping outlets, personal care facilities, medical clinics, administrative offices, finance and navigation offices, ship-to-shore communications systems, and the cargo hold, from the manifest to the unmanifest, from particle to wave, transmuting to a neutral energy. Clearing all EMF energy fluctuations from solar flares and geomagnetic storms, cellular transmissions, and all forms of radiation, in matter, dark matter, antimatter, energy, space, time, and all alternate realities, mind control, non-beneficial interdimensional beings, earthbound tricksters, extraterrestrials, artificial intelligence, subliminal messages, hypnosis and posthypnotic suggestions in all forms, collective-consciousness fear, anxiety, trauma, emotional charges, cords, attachments, implants, hooks, entities, and thought forms, seen or unseen, cloaked or uncloaked, in conscious, subconscious, and all altered states of consciousness, even

if they are changing frequencies and dimensions, simultaneously, in matter, dark matter, antimatter, energy, space, time, and all alternate realities. We are moving everything into the containment orb at the count of 10.

1, 2, 3, 4, 5, 6, 7, 8, 9, 10 - Increasing the cohesion to the 987th Fibonacci number.

We are clearing all imprints, echoes, residuals, energetic tattoos associated with what we just cleared, simultaneously, in matter, dark matter, antimatter, energy, space, time, and all alternate realities. We are moving everything into the containment orb at the count of 10.

1, 2, 3, 4, 5, 6, 7, 8, 9, 10 - Increasing the cohesion to the 987th Fibonacci number.

↷ (Projecting) We are sealing the containment orb.

↶ (Extracting) Sending it to the Central Sun.

And so it is, and so it is, and so it is.

INTERCITY BUS AND TRAIN

☽ (Projecting) We are placing _____(Bus/Train Route/Name) in an orb with mirrors facing in and mirrors facing out, the Sirius B Council on the outside, Archangels Raphael, Uriel, Gabriel, and Michael at the four cardinal points.

We are placing a containment orb to the right of the main orb with mirrors facing in and mirrors facing out, the Sirius B Council on the outside, Archangels Raphael, Uriel, Gabriel, and Michael at the four cardinal points.

We invoke all the Ascended Masters and Angelic Beings of the Universe to go up as a conduit, through the Galactic Core, Central Sun, Secret Sun, Platinum Sun, in conscious, subconscious, and all altered states of consciousness, and go down into the _____ (Bus/Train Route/Name).

☾ (Extracting) We are clearing _____(Bus/Train Route/Name), the driver(s), passenger(s), crew members and animals traveling in the _____(Bus/Train Route/Name); we are clearing the passenger compartment, including tray tables, overhead bins, carry-on baggage, seats, entertainment systems, individual seat controls, carpets, lavatories (if any), and all other furniture, fixtures and galleys (if applicable), as well as the storage compartments, from the manifest to the unmanifest, from particle to wave, transmuting to a neutral energy. Clearing all EMF energy fluctuations from solar flares and geomagnetic storms, cellular transmissions, and all forms of radiation, in matter, dark matter, antimatter, energy, space, time, and all alternate realities, mind control, non-beneficial interdimensional beings, earthbound tricksters, extraterrestrials, artificial intelligence, subliminal messages, hypnosis and posthypnotic suggestions in all forms, collective-consciousness fear, anxiety, trauma, emotional charges, cords, attachments, implants, hooks, entities, and thought forms, seen or unseen, cloaked or uncloaked, in conscious, subconscious, and all altered states of consciousness, even

if they are changing frequencies and dimensions, simultaneously, in matter, dark matter, antimatter, energy, space, time, and all alternate realities. We are moving everything into the containment orb at the count of 10.

1, 2, 3, 4, 5, 6, 7, 8, 9, 10 - Increasing the cohesion to the 987th Fibonacci number.

We are clearing all imprints, echoes, residuals, energetic tattoos associated with what we just cleared, simultaneously, in matter, dark matter, antimatter, energy, space, time, and all alternate realities. We are moving everything into the containment orb at the count of 10.

1, 2, 3, 4, 5, 6, 7, 8, 9, 10 - Increasing the cohesion to the 987th Fibonacci number.

↷ (Projecting) We are sealing the containment orb.

↶ (Extracting) Sending it to the Central Sun.

And so it is, and so it is, and so it is.

LOCAL BUS

☽ (Projecting) We are placing _____(Name of Bus Route) in an orb with mirrors facing in and mirrors facing out, the Sirius B Council on the outside, Archangels Raphael, Uriel, Gabriel, and Michael at the four cardinal points.

We are placing a containment orb to the right of the main orb with mirrors facing in and mirrors facing out, the Sirius B Council on the outside, Archangels Raphael, Uriel, Gabriel, and Michael at the four cardinal points.

We invoke all the Ascended Masters and Angelic Beings of the Universe to go up as a conduit, through the Galactic Core, Central Sun, Secret Sun, Platinum Sun, in conscious, subconscious, and all altered states of consciousness, and go down into the _____ (Name of Bus Route).

☾ (Extracting) We are clearing all negative energy in the bus, the bus driver, the collector, all passenger(s) traveling in the _____ (Name of Bus Route) the bus and the passenger compartment, including carry-on baggage, seating, flooring, and all other built-in fixtures, from the manifest to the unmanifest, from particle to wave, transmuting to a neutral energy. Clearing all EMF energy fluctuations from solar flares and geomagnetic storms, cellular transmissions, and all forms of radiation, in matter, dark matter, antimatter, energy, space, time, and all alternate realities, mind control, non-beneficial interdimensional beings, earthbound tricksters, extraterrestrials, artificial intelligence, subliminal messages, hypnosis and posthypnotic suggestions in all forms, collective-consciousness fear, anxiety, trauma, emotional charges, cords, attachments, implants, hooks, entities, and thought forms, seen or unseen, cloaked or uncloaked, in conscious, subconscious, and all altered states of consciousness, even if they are changing frequencies and dimensions, simultaneously, in matter, dark matter, antimatter, energy, space, time, and all alternate

realities. We are moving everything into the containment orb at the count of 10.

1, 2, 3, 4, 5, 6, 7, 8, 9, 10 - Increasing the cohesion to the 987th Fibonacci number.

We are clearing all imprints, echoes, residuals, energetic tattoos associated with what we just cleared, simultaneously, in matter, dark matter, antimatter, energy, space, time, and all alternate realities. We are moving everything into the containment orb at the count of 10.

1, 2, 3, 4, 5, 6, 7, 8, 9, 10 - Increasing the cohesion to the 987th Fibonacci number.

◠ (Projecting) We are sealing the containment orb.

◡ (Extracting) Sending it to the Central Sun.

◠ (Projecting) We invoke all of the Ascended Masters and Angelic Beings of the Universe to go up as a conduit, through the Galactic Core, Central Sun, Secret Sun, Platinum Sun in conscious, subconscious, and all altered states of consciousness, and, taking Ruby Red light and eucalyptus saplings, go down through the bus itself and all the people on the bus to the center of the New Earth, the crystal core of the Mother, completely grounding the bus and people on the bus.

And so it is, and so it is, and so it is.

PASSENGER CAR
OR TRUCK

↻ (Projecting) We are placing the vehicle in an orb with mirrors facing in and mirrors facing out, the Sirius B Council on the outside, Archangels Raphael, Uriel, Gabriel, and Michael at the four cardinal points.

We are placing a containment orb to the right of the main orb with mirrors facing in and mirrors facing out, the Sirius B Council on the outside, Archangels Raphael, Uriel, Gabriel, and Michael at the four cardinal points.

We invoke all the Ascended Masters and Angelic Beings of the Universe to go up as a conduit, in conscious, through the Galactic Core, Central Sun, Secret Sun, Platinum Sun, in conscious, subconscious, and all altered states of consciousness, and then to go down into the vehicle.

◠ (Extracting) We are clearing the vehicle, including all passengers, seating, electronic consoles, individual seat controls, carpets, and all other personal property such as cellphones, tablets, laptops, GPS, or other devices, from the manifest to the unmanifest, from particle to wave, transmuting to a neutral energy. Clearing all EMF energy fluctuations from solar flares and geomagnetic storms, cellular transmissions, and all forms of radiation, in matter, dark matter, antimatter, energy, space, time, and all alternate realities, mind control, non-beneficial interdimensional beings, earthbound tricksters, extraterrestrials, artificial intelligence, subliminal messages, hypnosis and posthypnotic suggestions in all forms, collective-consciousness fear, anxiety, trauma, emotional charges, cords, attachments, implants, hooks, entities, and thought forms, seen or unseen, cloaked or uncloaked, in conscious, subconscious, and all altered states of consciousness, even if they are changing frequencies and dimensions, simultaneously, in matter, dark matter, antimatter, energy, space, time, and all alternate realities. We are moving everything into the containment orb at the count of 10.

1, 2, 3, 4, 5, 6, 7, 8, 9, 10 - Increasing the cohesion to the 987th Fibonacci number.

We are clearing all imprints, echoes, residuals, energetic tattoos associated with what we just cleared, simultaneously, in matter, dark matter, antimatter, energy, space, time, and all alternate realities. We are moving everything into the containment orb at the count of 10.

1, 2, 3, 4, 5, 6, 7, 8, 9, 10 - Increasing the cohesion to the 987th Fibonacci number.

↷ (Projecting) We are sealing the containment orb.

↶ (Extracting) Sending it to the Central Sun.

And so it is, and so it is, and so it is.

RENTAL CARS

↻ (Projecting) We are placing the rental vehicle and _____ (Name of renter) in an orb with mirrors facing in and mirrors facing out, the Sirius B Council on the outside, Archangels Raphael, Uriel, Gabriel, and Michael at the four cardinal points.

We are placing a containment orb to the right of the main orb with mirrors facing in and mirrors facing out, the Sirius B Council on the outside, Archangels Raphael, Uriel, Gabriel, and Michael at the four cardinal points.

We invoke all the Ascended Masters and Angelic Beings of the Universe to go up as a conduit, through the Galactic Core, Central Sun, Secret Sun, Platinum Sun, into conscious, subconscious, and all altered states of consciousness, and then to go down into the vehicle.

↻ (Extracting) We are clearing the rental vehicle and _____ (Name of renter) and drivers and passengers traveling together with the renter, all previous drivers, passengers, and animals who have traveled in the vehicle, all seating, electronic consoles, individual seat controls, carpets, and all other personal property including GPS or other electronic devices, from the manifest to the unmanifest, from particle to wave, transmuting to a neutral energy. Clearing all EMF energy fluctuations from solar flares and geomagnetic storms, cellular transmissions, and all forms of radiation, in matter, dark matter, antimatter, energy, space, time, and all alternate realities, mind control, non-beneficial interdimensional beings, earthbound tricksters, extraterrestrials, artificial intelligence, subliminal messages, hypnosis and posthypnotic suggestions in all forms, collective-consciousness fear, anxiety, trauma, emotional charges, cords, attachments, implants, hooks, entities, and thought forms, seen or unseen, cloaked or uncloaked, in conscious, subconscious, and all altered states of consciousness, even if they are changing frequencies and dimensions, simultaneously, in matter, dark matter, antimatter,

energy, space, time, and all alternate realities. We are moving everything into the containment orb at the count of 10.

1, 2, 3, 4, 5, 6, 7, 8, 9, 10 - Increasing the cohesion to the 987th Fibonacci number.

We are clearing all imprints, echoes, residuals, energetic tattoos associated with what we just cleared, simultaneously, in matter, dark matter, antimatter, energy, space, time, and all alternate realities. We are moving everything into the containment orb at the count of 10.

1, 2, 3, 4, 5, 6, 7, 8, 9, 10 - Increasing the cohesion to the 987th Fibonacci number.

☽ (Projecting) We are sealing the containment orb.

☾ (Extracting) Sending it to the Central Sun.

And so it is, and so it is, and so it is

RIDESHARES/TAXIS

◗ (Projecting) We are placing the vehicle transporting _____ (Name) in an orb with mirrors facing in and mirrors facing out, the Sirius B Council on the outside, Archangels Raphael, Uriel, Gabriel, and Michael at the four cardinal points.

We are placing a containment orb to the right of the main orb with mirrors facing in and mirrors facing out, the Sirius B Council on the outside, Archangels Raphael, Uriel, Gabriel, and Michael at the four cardinal points.

We invoke all the Ascended Masters and Angelic Beings of the Universe to go up as a conduit, through the Galactic Core, Central Sun, Secret Sun, Platinum Sun, into conscious, subconscious, and all altered states of consciousness, and then to go down into the vehicle transporting _____(Name).

◖ (Extracting) We are clearing _____(Name) and the rideshare/taxi vehicle, including all previous drivers, passengers and animals who have traveled in the vehicle, all seating, electronic consoles, individual seat controls, carpet, and all other personal property such as cellphones, tablets, laptops, GPS, or other devices, from the manifest to the unmanifest, from particle to wave, transmuting to a neutral energy. Clearing all EMF energy fluctuations from solar flares and geomagnetic storms, cellular transmissions, and all forms of radiation, in matter, dark matter, antimatter, energy, space, time, and all alternate realities, mind control, non-beneficial interdimensional beings, earthbound tricksters, extraterrestrials, artificial intelligence, subliminal messages, hypnosis and posthypnotic suggestions in all forms, collective-consciousness fear, anxiety, trauma, emotional charges, cords, attachments, implants, hooks, entities, and thought forms, seen or unseen, cloaked or uncloaked, in conscious, subconscious, and all altered states of consciousness, even if they are changing frequencies and dimensions, simultaneously, in matter, dark matter, antimatter, energy, space, time, and all alternate

realities. We are moving everything into the containment orb at the count of 10.

1, 2, 3, 4, 5, 6, 7, 8, 9, 10 - Increasing the cohesion to the 987th Fibonacci number.

We are clearing all imprints, echoes, residuals, energetic tattoos associated with what we just cleared, simultaneously, in matter, dark matter, antimatter, energy, space, time, and all alternate realities. We are moving everything into the containment orb at the count of 10.

1, 2, 3, 4, 5, 6, 7, 8, 9, 10 - Increasing the cohesion to the 987th Fibonacci number.

↷ (Projecting) We are sealing the containment orb.

↶ (Extracting) Sending it to the Central Sun.

And so it is, and so it is, and so it is.

TRANSPORTATION TERMINALS

↷ (Projecting) We are placing _____(Transportation Facility) in an orb with mirrors facing in and mirrors facing out, the Sirius B Council on the outside, Archangels Raphael, Uriel, Gabriel, and Michael at the four cardinal points.

We are placing a containment orb to the right of the main orb with mirrors facing in and mirrors facing out, the Sirius B Council on the outside, Archangels Raphael, Uriel, Gabriel, and Michael at the four cardinal points.

We invoke all the Ascended Masters and Angelic Beings of the Universe to go up as a conduit, through the Galactic Core, Central Sun, Secret Sun, Platinum Sun, into conscious, subconscious, and all altered states of consciousness, and then to go down into the _____(Transportation Facility).

↻ (Extracting) We are clearing _____(Transportation Facility), including all passengers, friends, family, and business associates seeing them off, all crew members, food service locations, retail stores, taxi drivers, security and facility management personnel, all other transportation workers and animals, from the manifest to the unmanifest, from particle to wave, transmuting to a neutral energy. Clearing all EMF energy fluctuations from solar flares and geomagnetic storms, cellular transmissions, and all forms of radiation, in matter, dark matter, antimatter, energy, space, time, and all alternate realities, mind control, non-beneficial interdimensional beings, earthbound tricksters, extraterrestrials, artificial intelligence, subliminal messages, hypnosis and posthypnotic suggestions in all forms, collective-consciousness fear, anxiety, trauma, emotional charges, cords, attachments, implants, hooks, entities, and thought forms, seen or unseen, cloaked or uncloaked, in conscious, subconscious, and all altered states of consciousness, even if they are changing frequencies and dimensions, simultaneously, in matter, dark matter, antimatter, energy, space, time, and all alternate realities. We are moving everything into the containment orb at the count of 10.

1, 2, 3, 4, 5, 6, 7, 8, 9, 10 - Increasing the cohesion to the 987th Fibonacci number.

We are clearing all imprints, echoes, residuals, energetic tattoos associated with what we just cleared, simultaneously, in matter, dark matter, antimatter, energy, space, time, and all alternate realities. We are moving everything into the containment orb at the count of 10.

1, 2, 3, 4, 5, 6, 7, 8, 9, 10 - Increasing the cohesion to the 987th Fibonacci number.

↷ (Projecting) We are sealing the containment orb.

↶ (Extracting) Sending it to the Central Sun.

And so it is, and so it is, and so it is.

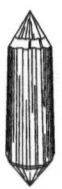

CHAPTER 9

EARTH CHANGES

GEOMAGNETIC STORMS

☽ (Projecting) We are placing _____(Name) in an orb with mirrors facing in and mirrors facing out, the Sirius B Council on the outside, Archangels Raphael, Uriel, Gabriel, and Michael at the four cardinal points.

We are placing a containment orb to the right of the main orb with mirrors facing in and mirrors facing out, the Sirius B Council on the outside, Archangels Raphael, Uriel, Gabriel, and Michael at the four cardinal points.

We are facilitating the incoming download of enlightenment and spiritual light code that is being transmitted by the Geomagnetic Storms into _____(Name), and we invoke all the Ascended Masters and Angelic Beings of the Universe, to go up as a conduit, through the Galactic Core, Central Sun, Secret Sun, Platinum Sun, into conscious, subconscious, and all altered states of consciousness, and down into _____(Name).

☾ (Extracting) We are clearing all radiation and non-beneficial energy coming from the Geomagnetic Storms that is causing fear, anxiety, and trauma and over-energizing the physical body, and we are preventing any radiation or harmful energy from entering _____(Name) auric field, from the manifest to the unmanifest, from particle to wave, transmuting to a neutral energy. Clearing all EMF energy fluctuations from solar flares and geomagnetic storms, cellular transmissions, and all forms of radiation, in matter, dark matter, antimatter, energy, space, time, and all alternate realities, mind control, non-beneficial interdimensional beings, earthbound tricksters, extraterrestrials, artificial intelligence, subliminal messages, hypnosis and posthypnotic suggestions in all forms, collective-consciousness fear, anxiety, trauma, emotional charges, cords, attachments, implants, hooks, entities, and thought forms, seen or unseen, cloaked or uncloaked, in conscious, subconscious, and all altered states of consciousness, even if they are changing frequencies and dimensions, simultaneously, in matter, dark matter, antimatter, energy, space, time, and all alternative realities. We are moving everything into the containment orb at the count of 10.

1, 2, 3, 4, 5, 6, 7, 8, 9, 10 - Increasing the cohesion to the 987th Fibonacci number.

We are clearing all imprints, echoes, residuals, energetic tattoos associated with what we just cleared, simultaneously, in matter, dark matter, antimatter, energy, space, time, and all alternate realities. We are moving everything into the containment orb at the count of 10.

1, 2, 3, 4, 5, 6, 7, 8, 9, 10 - Increasing the cohesion to the 987th Fibonacci number.

↷ (Projecting) We are sealing the containment orb.

↶ (Extracting) Sending it to the Central Sun.

And so it is, and so it is, and so it is.

SCHUMANN RESONANCE SPIKES

↻ (Projecting) We are placing _____(Name) in an orb with mirrors facing in and mirrors facing out, the Sirius B Council on the outside, Archangels Raphael, Uriel, Gabriel, and Michael at the four cardinal points.

We are placing a containment orb to the right of the main orb with mirrors facing in and mirrors facing out, the Sirius B Council on the outside, Archangels Raphael, Uriel, Gabriel, and Michael at the four cardinal points.

We are facilitating the incoming download of enlightenment and spiritual light code that is being transmitted by the Schumann Resonance spikes into _____(Name).

We invoke all the Ascended Masters and Angelic Beings of the Universe to go up as a conduit, through the Galactic Core, Central Sun, Secret Sun, Platinum Sun, into conscious, subconscious, and all altered states of consciousness, and down into _____(Name).

↺ (Extracting) We are clearing all radiation and energy coming from the Schumann Resonance spikes that is causing fear, anxiety, and trauma and over-energizing and shocking the physical body, and we are clearing any harmful planetary energy and radiation, from the manifest to the unmanifest, from particle to wave, transmuting to a neutral energy. Clearing all EMF energy fluctuations from solar flares and geomagnetic storms, cellular transmissions, and all forms of radiation, in matter, dark matter, antimatter, energy, space, time, and all alternate realities, mind control, non-beneficial interdimensional beings, earthbound tricksters, extraterrestrials, artificial intelligence, subliminal messages, hypnosis and posthypnotic suggestions in all forms, collective-consciousness fear, anxiety, trauma, emotional charges, cords, attachments, implants, hooks, entities, and thought forms, seen or unseen, cloaked or uncloaked, in conscious, subconscious, and all altered states of consciousness, even if they are changing frequencies and dimensions, simultaneously, in matter, dark matter, antimatter, energy, space, time, and all alternative realities. We are moving everything into the containment orb at the count of 10.

1, 2, 3, 4, 5, 6, 7, 8, 9, 10 - Increasing the cohesion to the 987th Fibonacci number.

We are clearing all imprints, echoes, residuals, energetic tattoos associated with what we just cleared, simultaneously, in matter, dark matter, antimatter, energy, space, time, and all alternate realities. We are moving everything into the containment orb at the count of 10.

1, 2, 3, 4, 5, 6, 7, 8, 9, 10 - Increasing the cohesion to the 987th Fibonacci number.

☽ (Projecting) We are sealing the containment orb.

☾ (Extracting) Sending it to the Central Sun.

And so it is, and so it is, and so it is.

SOLAR FLARES

☽ (Projecting) We are placing _____(Name) in an orb with mirrors facing in and mirrors facing out, the Sirius B Council on the outside, Archangels Raphael, Uriel, Gabriel, and Michael at the four cardinal points.

We are placing a containment orb to the right of the main orb with mirrors facing in and mirrors facing out, the Sirius B Council on the outside, Archangels Raphael, Uriel, Gabriel, and Michael at the four cardinal points.

We are facilitating the incoming download of enlightenment and spiritual light code that is being transmitted by the Solar Flares into _____(Name).

We invoke all the Ascended Masters and Angelic Beings of the Universe to go up as a conduit, through the Galactic Core, Central Sun, Secret Sun, Platinum Sun, into conscious, subconscious, and all altered states of consciousness, and down into _____(Name).

☾ (Extracting) We are clearing the Solar Flare's radiation and energy, which is causing fear, anxiety, and trauma and shocking the physical body with harmful energy, and preventing it from entering _____(Name) auric field, from the manifest to the unmanifest, from particle to wave, transmuting to a neutral energy. Clearing all EMF energy fluctuations from solar flares and geomagnetic storms, cellular transmissions, and all forms of radiation, in matter, dark matter, antimatter, energy, space, time, and all alternate realities, mind control, non-beneficial interdimensional beings, earthbound tricksters, extraterrestrials, artificial intelligence, subliminal messages, hypnosis and posthypnotic suggestions in all forms, collective-consciousness fear, anxiety, trauma, emotional charges, cords, attachments, implants, hooks, entities, and thought forms, seen or unseen, cloaked or uncloaked, in conscious, subconscious, and all altered states of consciousness, even if they are changing frequencies and dimensions, simultaneously, in matter, dark matter, antimatter, energy, space, time, and all alternative realities. We are moving everything into the containment orb at the count of 10.

1, 2, 3, 4, 5, 6, 7, 8, 9, 10 - Increasing the cohesion to the 987th Fibonacci number.

We are clearing all imprints, echoes, residuals, energetic tattoos associated with what we just cleared, simultaneously, in matter, dark matter, antimatter, energy, space, time, and all alternate realities. We are moving everything into the containment orb at the count of 10.

1, 2, 3, 4, 5, 6, 7, 8, 9, 10 - Increasing the cohesion to the 987th Fibonacci number.

☽ (Projecting) We are sealing the containment orb.

☾ (Extracting) Sending it to the Central Sun.

And so it is, and so it is, and so it is.

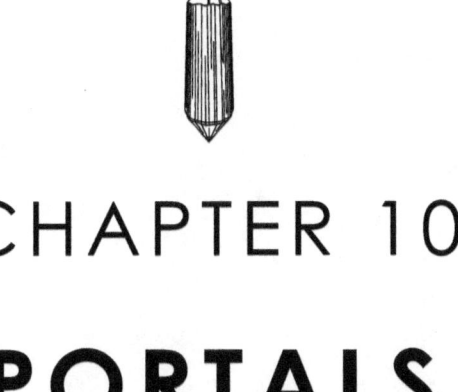

CHAPTER 10

PORTALS

OPENING A PORTAL

↻ (Projecting) We are placing _____(Portal Location) to an orb with mirrors facing in and mirrors facing out, the Sirius B Council on the outside, Archangels Raphael, Uriel, Gabriel, and Michael at the four cardinal points.

We are placing a containment orb to the right of the main orb with mirrors facing in and mirrors facing out, the Sirius B Council on the outside, Archangels Raphael, Uriel, Gabriel, and Michael at the four cardinal points.

We invoke all the Ascended Masters and Angelic Beings of the Universe to go up as a conduit, through the Galactic Core, Central Sun, Secret Sun, Platinum Sun, into conscious, subconscious, and all altered states of consciousness, and down into _____(Portal Location)

☊ (Extracting) We are clearing _____(Portal Location), from the manifest to the unmanifest, from particle to wave, transmuting to a neutral energy. Clearing all EMF energy fluctuations from solar flares and geomagnetic storms, cellular transmissions, and all forms of radiation, in matter, dark matter, antimatter, energy, space, time, and all alternate realities, mind control, non-beneficial interdimensional beings, earthbound tricksters, extraterrestrials, artificial intelligence, subliminal messages, hypnosis and posthypnotic suggestions in all forms, collective-consciousness fear, anxiety, trauma, emotional charges, cords, attachments, implants, hooks, entities, and thought forms, seen or unseen, cloaked or uncloaked, in conscious, subconscious, and all altered states of consciousness, even if they are changing frequencies and dimensions, simultaneously, in matter, dark matter, antimatter, energy, space, time, and all alternative realities. We are moving everything into the containment orb at the count of 10.

1, 2, 3, 4, 5, 6, 7, 8, 9, 10 - Increasing the cohesion to the 987th Fibonacci number.

We are clearing all imprints, echoes, residuals, energetic tattoos associated with what we just cleared, simultaneously, in matter, dark matter, antimatter, energy, space, time, and all alternate realities. We are moving everything into the containment orb at the count of 10.

1, 2, 3, 4, 5, 6, 7, 8, 9, 10 - Increasing the cohesion to the 987th Fibonacci number.

☽ (Projecting) We are sealing the containment orb.

☾ (Extracting) Sending it to the Central Sun.

☽ (Projecting) We are opening the _____(Portal location).

And so it is, and so it is, and so it is.

SHUTTING A PORTAL

◯ (Projecting) We are placing _____(Portal Location) in an orb with mirrors facing in and mirrors facing out, the Sirius B Council on the outside, Archangels Raphael, Uriel, Gabriel, and Michael at the four cardinal points.

We are placing a containment orb to the right of the main orb with mirrors facing in and mirrors facing out, the Sirius B Council on the outside, Archangels Raphael, Uriel, Gabriel, and Michael at the four cardinal points.

We invoke all of the Ascended Masters and Angelic Beings of the Universe to go up as a conduit, through the Galactic Core, Central Sun, Secret Sun, Platinum Sun, into conscious, subconscious, and all altered states of consciousness, and down into _____(Portal Location).

◯ (Extracting) We are clearing _____(Portal Location) of all emotional charges and energy, from the manifest to the unmanifest, from particle to wave, transmuting to a neutral energy. Clearing all EMF energy fluctuations from solar flares and geomagnetic storms, high speed cellular radiation, cellular transmissions, and all forms of radiation, in matter, dark matter, antimatter, energy, space, time, and all alternate realities, mind control, non-beneficial interdimensional beings, earthbound tricksters, extraterrestrials, artificial intelligence, subliminal messages, hypnosis and posthypnotic suggestions in all forms, collective-consciousness fear, anxiety, trauma, emotional charges, cords, attachments, implants, hooks, entities, and thought forms, seen or unseen, cloaked or uncloaked, in conscious, subconscious, and all altered states of consciousness, even if they are changing frequencies and dimensions, simultaneously, in matter, dark matter, antimatter, energy, space, time, and all alternative realities. We are moving everything into the containment orb at the count of 10.

1, 2, 3, 4, 5, 6, 7, 8, 9, 10 - Increasing the cohesion to the 987th Fibonacci number.

We are clearing all imprints, echoes, residuals, energetic tattoos associated with what we just cleared, simultaneously, in matter, dark matter, antimatter, energy, space, time, and all alternate realities. We are moving everything into the containment orb at the count of 10.

1, 2, 3, 4, 5, 6, 7, 8, 9, 10 - Increasing the cohesion to the 987th Fibonacci number.

↷ (Projecting) We are sealing the containment orb.

↶ (Extracting) Sending it to the Central Sun.

↷ (Projecting) We are invoking the Ascended Masters and Angelic Beings to go up as a conduit, through the Galactic Core, Central Sun, Secret Sun, Platinum Sun, into conscious, subconscious, and all altered states of consciousness, and go down into _____(Portal Location), closing and sealing the portal now.

And so it is, and so it is, and so it is.

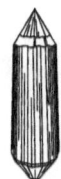

CHAPTER 11

MINERALS

CHARGING MINERALS

☽ (Projecting) We are placing _____(Name of Mineral) in an orb with mirrors facing in and mirrors facing out, the Sirius B Council on the outside, Archangels Raphael, Uriel, Gabriel, and Michael at the four cardinal points.

We invoke all the Ascended Masters and Angelic Beings of the Universe to go up as a conduit, through the Galactic Core, Central Sun, Secret Sun, Platinum Sun, into conscious, subconscious, and all altered states of consciousness, and down into _____(Name of Mineral).

We are charging _____(Name of Mineral) with celestial sunlight and lunar moonlight; Galactic Gold, Electric Ultra Violet Blue, Platinum, and Plasma light code; Christ chambers; and the Atlantis crystal array Violet Flame, raising the vibration and frequency of the _____(Name of Mineral) to the highest level at which it can vibrate.

And so it is, and so it is, and so it is.

CLEARING MINERALS

☽ (Projecting) We are placing _____(Name of Mineral) in an orb with mirrors facing in and mirrors facing out, the Sirius B Council on the outside, Archangels Raphael, Uriel, Gabriel, and Michael at the four cardinal points.

We are placing a containment orb to the right of the main orb with mirrors facing in and mirrors facing out, the Sirius B Council on the outside, Archangels Raphael, Uriel, Gabriel, and Michael at the four cardinal points.

We invoke all the Ascended Masters and Angelic Beings of the Universe to go up as a conduit, through the Galactic Core, Central Sun, Secret Sun, Platinum Sun, into conscious, subconscious, and all altered states of consciousness, and down into _____(Name of Mineral).

☽ (Extracting) We are energetically clearing the _____(Name of Mineral) of everything it has recorded and absorbed, emotional charges, from the manifest to the unmanifest, from particle to wave, transmuting to a neutral energy. Clearing all EMF energy fluctuations from solar flares and geomagnetic storms, cellular transmissions, and all forms of radiation, in matter, dark matter, antimatter, energy, space, time, and all alternate realities, mind control, non-beneficial interdimensional beings, earthbound tricksters, extraterrestrials, artificial intelligence, subliminal messages, hypnosis and posthypnotic suggestions in all forms, collective-consciousness fear, anxiety, trauma, emotional charges, cords, attachments, implants, hooks, entities, and thought forms, seen or unseen, cloaked or uncloaked, in conscious, subconscious, and all altered states of consciousness, even if they are changing frequencies and dimensions, simultaneously, in matter, dark matter, antimatter, energy, space, time, and all alternative realities. We are moving everything into the containment orb at the count of 10.

1, 2, 3, 4, 5, 6, 7, 8, 9, 10 - Increasing the cohesion to the 987th Fibonacci number.

We are clearing all imprints, echoes, residuals, energetic tattoos associated with what we just cleared, simultaneously, in matter, dark matter, antimatter, energy, space, time, and all alternate realities. We are moving everything into the containment orb at the count of 10.

1, 2, 3, 4, 5, 6, 7, 8, 9, 10 - Increasing the cohesion to the 987th Fibonacci number.

☾ (Projecting) We are sealing the containment orb.

☾ (Extracting) Sending it to the Central Sun.

And so it is, and so it is, and so it is.

PROJECTING MINERALS

↻ (Projecting) We are placing _____(Name of Mineral) in an orb with mirrors facing in and mirrors facing out, the Sirius B Council on the outside, Archangels Raphael, Uriel, Gabriel, and Michael at the four cardinal points.

We invoke all the Ascended Masters and Angelic Beings of the Universe to go up as a conduit, through the Galactic Core, Central Sun, Secret Sun, Platinum Sun, into conscious, subconscious, and all altered states of consciousness, and down into _____(Name of Mineral).

We are projecting and channeling the _____(Name of Mineral) to _____(Destination).

And so it is, and so it is, and so it is.

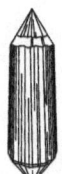

CHAPTER 12

POSSESSIONS

ALCOHOL ENTITIES

◯ (Projecting) We are placing _____(Name) in an orb with mirrors facing in and mirrors facing out, the Sirius B Council on the outside, Archangels Raphael, Uriel, Gabriel, and Michael at the four cardinal points.

We are placing a containment orb to the right of the main orb with mirrors facing in and mirrors facing out, the Sirius B Council on the outside, Archangels Raphael, Uriel, Gabriel, and Michael at the four cardinal points.

We invoke all the Ascended Masters and Angelic Beings of the Universe to go up as a conduit, through the Galactic Core, Central Sun, Secret Sun, Platinum Sun, into conscious, subconscious, and all altered states of consciousness, and down into _____(Name).

◯ (Extracting) We are clearing _____(Name) of all alcohol entities, alcohol-related projected energy, and alcohol attachments, from the manifest to the unmanifest, from particle to wave, transmuting to a neutral energy. Clearing all EMF energy fluctuations from solar flares and geomagnetic storms, cellular transmissions, and all forms of radiation, in matter, dark matter, antimatter, energy, space, time, and all alternate realities, mind control, non-beneficial interdimensional beings, earthbound tricksters, extraterrestrials, artificial intelligence, subliminal messages, hypnosis and posthypnotic suggestions in all forms, collective-consciousness fear, anxiety, trauma, emotional charges, cords, attachments, implants, hooks, entities, and thought forms, seen or unseen, cloaked or uncloaked, in conscious, subconscious, and all altered states of consciousness, even if they are changing frequencies and dimensions, simultaneously, in matter, dark matter, antimatter, energy, space, time, and all alternative realities. We are moving everything into the containment orb at the count of 10.

1, 2, 3, 4, 5, 6, 7, 8, 9, 10 - Increasing the cohesion to the 987th Fibonacci number.

We are clearing all imprints, echoes, residuals, energetic tattoos associated with what we just cleared, simultaneously, in matter, dark matter, antimatter, energy, space, time, and all alternate realities. We are moving everything into the containment orb at the count of 10.

1, 2, 3, 4, 5, 6, 7, 8, 9, 10 - Increasing the cohesion to the 987th Fibonacci number.

◯ (Projecting) We are sealing the containment orb.

◯ (Extracting) Sending it to the Central Sun.

And so it is, and so it is, and so it is.

DEMONIC

◔ (Projecting) We are placing _____(Name) in an orb with mirrors facing in and mirrors facing out, the Sirius B Council on the outside, Archangels Raphael, Uriel, Gabriel, and Michael at the four cardinal points.

We are placing a containment orb to the right of the main orb with mirrors facing in and mirrors facing out, the Sirius B Council on the outside, Archangels Raphael, Uriel, Gabriel, and Michael at the four cardinal points.

We invoke all the Ascended Masters and Angelic Beings of the Universe to go up as a conduit, through the Galactic Core, Central Sun, Secret Sun, Platinum Sun, into conscious, subconscious, and all altered states of consciousness, and down into _____(Name).

◖ (Extracting) We are clearing _____(Name) of all demonic predators, demonic projected energy, and demonic attachments, from the manifest to the unmanifest, from particle to wave, transmuting to a neutral energy. Clearing all EMF energy fluctuations from solar flares and geomagnetic storms, cellular transmissions, and all forms of radiation, in matter, dark matter, antimatter, energy, space, time, and all alternate realities, mind control, non-beneficial interdimensional beings, earthbound tricksters, extraterrestrials, artificial intelligence, subliminal messages, hypnosis and posthypnotic suggestions in all forms, collective-consciousness fear, anxiety, trauma, emotional charges, cords, attachments, implants, hooks, entities, and thought forms, seen or unseen, cloaked or uncloaked, in conscious, subconscious, and all altered states of consciousness, even if they are changing frequencies and dimensions, simultaneously, in matter, dark matter, antimatter, energy, space, time, and all alternative realities. We are moving everything into the containment orb at the count of 10.

1, 2, 3, 4, 5, 6, 7, 8, 9, 10 - Increasing the cohesion to the 987th Fibonacci number.

We are clearing all imprints, echoes, residuals, energetic tattoos associated with what we just cleared, simultaneously, in matter, dark matter, antimatter, energy, space, time, and all alternate realities. We are moving everything into the containment orb at the count of 10.

1, 2, 3, 4, 5, 6, 7, 8, 9, 10 - Increasing the cohesion to the 987th Fibonacci number.

↷ (Projecting) We are sealing the containment orb.

↶ (Extracting) Sending it to the Central Sun.

And so it is, and so it is, and so it is.

DRUG ADDICTION

↷ (Projecting) We are placing _____(Name) in an orb with mirrors facing in and mirrors facing out, the Sirius B Council on the outside, Archangels Raphael, Uriel, Gabriel, and Michael at the four cardinal points.

We are placing a containment orb to the right of the main orb with mirrors facing in and mirrors facing out, the Sirius B Council on the outside, Archangels Raphael, Uriel, Gabriel, and Michael at the four cardinal points.

We invoke all the Ascended Masters and Angelic Beings of the Universe to go up as a conduit, through the Galactic Core, Central Sun, Secret Sun, Platinum Sun, into conscious, subconscious, and all altered states of consciousness, and down into _____(Name).

↶ (Extracting) We are clearing _____(Name) of all drug-addiction possessions, emotionally charged drug-possession energy, and drug-possession attachments of all kinds, from the manifest to the unmanifest, from particle to wave, transmuting to a neutral energy. Clearing all EMF energy fluctuations from solar flares and geomagnetic storms, cellular transmissions, and all forms of radiation, in matter, dark matter, antimatter, energy, space, time, and all alternate realities, mind control, non-beneficial interdimensional beings, earthbound tricksters, extraterrestrials, artificial intelligence, subliminal messages, hypnosis and posthypnotic suggestions in all forms, collective-consciousness fear, anxiety, trauma, emotional charges, cords, attachments, implants, hooks, entities, and thought forms, seen or unseen, cloaked or uncloaked, in conscious, subconscious, and all altered states of consciousness, even if they are changing frequencies and dimensions, simultaneously, in matter, dark matter, antimatter, energy, space, time, and all alternative realities. We are moving everything into the containment orb at the count of 10.

1, 2, 3, 4, 5, 6, 7, 8, 9, 10 - Increasing the cohesion to the 987th Fibonacci number.

We are clearing all imprints, echoes, residuals, energetic tattoos associated with what we just cleared, simultaneously, in matter, dark matter, antimatter, energy, space, time, and all alternate realities. We are moving everything into the containment orb at the count of 10.

1, 2, 3, 4, 5, 6, 7, 8, 9, 10 - Increasing the cohesion to the 987th Fibonacci number.

↷ (Projecting) We are sealing the containment orb.

↶ (Extracting) Sending it to the Central Sun.

And so it is, and so it is, and so it is.

GAMBLING

☽ (Projecting) We are placing _____(Name) in an orb with mirrors facing in and mirrors facing out, the Sirius B Council on the outside, Archangels Raphael, Uriel, Gabriel, and Michael at the four cardinal points.

We are placing a containment orb to the right of the main orb with mirrors facing in and mirrors facing out, the Sirius B Council on the outside, Archangels Raphael, Uriel, Gabriel, and Michael at the four cardinal points.

We invoke all the Ascended Masters and Angelic Beings of the Universe to go up as a conduit, through the Galactic Core, Central Sun, Secret Sun, Platinum Sun, into conscious, subconscious, and all altered states of consciousness, and down into _____(Name).

☾ (Extracting) We are clearing _____(Name) of the gambling possession, all gambling projected energy, and all gambling possession attachments, from the manifest to the unmanifest, from particle to wave, transmuting to a neutral energy. Clearing all EMF energy fluctuations from solar flares and geomagnetic storms, cellular transmissions, and all forms of radiation, in matter, dark matter, antimatter, energy, space, time, and all alternate realities, mind control, non-beneficial interdimensional beings, earthbound tricksters, extraterrestrials, artificial intelligence, subliminal messages, hypnosis and posthypnotic suggestions in all forms, collective-consciousness fear, anxiety, trauma, emotional charges, cords, attachments, implants, hooks, entities, and thought forms, seen or unseen, cloaked or uncloaked, in conscious, subconscious, and all altered states of consciousness, even if they are changing frequencies and dimensions, simultaneously, in matter, dark matter, antimatter, energy, space, time, and all alternative realities. We are moving everything into the containment orb at the count of 10.

1, 2, 3, 4, 5, 6, 7, 8, 9, 10 - Increasing the cohesion to the 987th Fibonacci number.

We are clearing all imprints, echoes, residuals, energetic tattoos associated with what we just cleared, simultaneously, in matter, dark matter, antimatter, energy, space, time, and all alternate realities. We are moving everything into the containment orb at the count of 10.

1, 2, 3, 4, 5, 6, 7, 8, 9, 10 - Increasing the cohesion to the 987th Fibonacci number.

☽ (Projecting) We are sealing the containment orb.

☽ (Extracting) Sending it to the Central Sun.

And so it is, and so it is, and so it is.

PSYCHIC ATTACKS

☌ (Projecting) We are placing _____(Name) in an orb with mirrors facing in and mirrors facing out, the Sirius B Council on the outside, Archangels Raphael, Uriel, Gabriel, and Michael at the four cardinal points.

We are placing a containment orb to the right of the main orb with mirrors facing in and mirrors facing out, the Sirius B Council on the outside, Archangels Raphael, Uriel, Gabriel, and Michael at the four cardinal points.

We invoke all the Ascended Masters and Angelic Beings of the Universe to go up as a conduit, through the Galactic Core, Central Sun, Secret Sun, Platinum Sun, into conscious, subconscious, and all altered states of consciousness, and down into _____(Name).

☽ (Extracting) We are clearing _____(Name) of the psychic attack, including the incarnate person initiating it, any third parties assisting and any spirits invoked from the spirit realms, from the manifest to the unmanifest, from particle to wave, transmuting to a neutral energy. Clearing all EMF energy fluctuations from solar flares and geomagnetic storms, cellular transmissions, and all forms of radiation, in matter, dark matter, antimatter, energy, space, time, and all alternate realities, mind control, non-beneficial interdimensional beings, earthbound tricksters, extraterrestrials, artificial intelligence, subliminal messages, hypnosis and posthypnotic suggestions in all forms, collective-consciousness fear, anxiety, trauma, emotional charges, cords, attachments, implants, hooks, entities, and thought forms, seen or unseen, cloaked or uncloaked, in conscious, subconscious, and all altered states of consciousness, even if they are changing frequencies and dimensions, simultaneously, in matter, dark matter, antimatter, energy, space, time, and all alternative realities. We are moving everything into the containment orb at the count of 10.

1, 2, 3, 4, 5, 6, 7, 8, 9, 10 - Increasing the cohesion to the 987th Fibonacci number.

We are clearing all imprints, echoes, residuals, energetic tattoos associated with what we just cleared, simultaneously, in matter, dark matter, antimatter, energy, space, time, and all alternate realities. We are moving everything into the containment orb at the count of 10.

1, 2, 3, 4, 5, 6, 7, 8, 9, 10 - Increasing the cohesion to the 987th Fibonacci number.

↱ (Projecting) We are sealing the containment orb.

↰ (Extracting) Sending it to the Central Sun.

And so it is, and so it is, and so it is.

SEXUAL PREDATORS

↻ (Projecting) We are placing _____(Name) in an orb with mirrors facing in and mirrors facing out, the Sirius B Council on the outside, Archangels Raphael, Uriel, Gabriel, and Michael at the four cardinal points.

We are placing a containment orb to the right of the main orb with mirrors facing in and mirrors facing out, the Sirius B Council on the outside, Archangels Raphael, Uriel, Gabriel, and Michael at the four cardinal points.

We invoke all the Ascended Masters and Angelic Beings of the Universe to go up as a conduit, through the Galactic Core, Central Sun, Secret Sun, Platinum Sun, into conscious, subconscious, and all altered states of consciousness, and down into _____(Name).

↻ (Extracting) We are clearing _____(Name) of all sexual predators, sexual projected energy, and sexual attachments, from the manifest to the unmanifest, from particle to wave, transmuting to a neutral energy. Clearing all EMF energy fluctuations from solar flares and geomagnetic storms, cellular transmissions, and all forms of radiation, in matter, dark matter, antimatter, energy, space, time, and all alternate realities, mind control, non-beneficial interdimensional beings, earthbound tricksters, extraterrestrials, artificial intelligence, subliminal messages, hypnosis and posthypnotic suggestions in all forms, collective-consciousness fear, anxiety, trauma, emotional charges, cords, attachments, implants, hooks, entities, and thought forms, seen or unseen, cloaked or uncloaked, in conscious, subconscious, and all altered states of consciousness, even if they are changing frequencies and dimensions, simultaneously, in matter, dark matter, antimatter, energy, space, time, and all alternative realities. We are moving everything into the containment orb at the count of 10.

1, 2, 3, 4, 5, 6, 7, 8, 9, 10 - Increasing the cohesion to the 987th Fibonacci number.

We are clearing all imprints, echoes, residuals, energetic tattoos associated with what we just cleared, simultaneously, in matter, dark matter, antimatter, energy, space, time, and all alternate realities. We are moving everything into the containment orb at the count of 10.

1, 2, 3, 4, 5, 6, 7, 8, 9, 10 - Increasing the cohesion to the 987th Fibonacci number.

☽ (Projecting) We are sealing the containment orb.

☾ (Extracting) Sending it to the Central Sun.

And so it is, and so it is, and so it is.

TOBACCO/NICOTINE

↷ (Projecting) We are placing _____(Name) in an orb with mirrors facing in and mirrors facing out, the Sirius B Council on the outside, Archangels Raphael, Uriel, Gabriel, and Michael at the four cardinal points.

We are placing a containment orb to the right of the main orb with mirrors facing in and mirrors facing out, the Sirius B Council on the outside, Archangels Raphael, Uriel, Gabriel, and Michael at the four cardinal points.

We invoke all the Ascended Masters and Angelic Beings of the Universe to go up as a conduit, through the Galactic Core, Central Sun, Secret Sun, Platinum Sun, into conscious, subconscious, and all altered states of consciousness, and down into _____(Name).

↶ (Extracting) We are clearing _____(Name) of all tobacco entities and demons, from the manifest to the unmanifest, from particle to wave, transmuting to a neutral energy. Clearing all EMF energy fluctuations from solar flares and geomagnetic storms, cellular transmissions, and all forms of radiation, in matter, dark matter, antimatter, energy, space, time, and all alternate realities, mind control, non-beneficial interdimensional beings, earthbound tricksters, extraterrestrials, artificial intelligence, subliminal messages, hypnosis and posthypnotic suggestions in all forms, collective-consciousness fear, anxiety, trauma, emotional charges, cords, attachments, implants, hooks, entities, and thought forms, seen or unseen, cloaked or uncloaked, in conscious, subconscious, and all altered states of consciousness, even if they are changing frequencies and dimensions, simultaneously, in matter, dark matter, antimatter, energy, space, time, and all alternative realities. We are moving everything into the containment orb at the count of 10.

1, 2, 3, 4, 5, 6, 7, 8, 9, 10 - Increasing the cohesion to the 987th Fibonacci number.

We are clearing all imprints, echoes, residuals, energetic tattoos associated with what we just cleared, simultaneously, in matter, dark matter, antimatter, energy, space, time, and all alternate realities. We are moving everything into the containment orb at the count of 10.

1, 2, 3, 4, 5, 6, 7, 8, 9, 10 - Increasing the cohesion to the 987th Fibonacci number.

☽ (Projecting) We are sealing the containment orb.

☾ (Extracting) Sending it to the Central Sun.

And so it is, and so it is, and so it is.

ABOUT THE AUTHOR

Paul Harry Simons is a spiritual medium who heals, teaches, and trains people from all walks of life in ways of moving energy to create better outcomes. For more info, please see MediumPaul.com

ABOUT THE PUBLISHER

The Sager Group was founded in 1984. In 2012 it was chartered as a multimedia content brand, with the intent of empowering those who create art—an umbrella beneath which makers can pursue, and profit from, their craft directly, without gatekeepers. TSG publishes books; ministers to artists and provides modest grants; and produces documentary, feature, and commercial films. By harnessing the means of production, The Sager Group helps artists help themselves. For more information, please see TheSagerGroup.net.

MORE BOOKS FROM THE SAGER GROUP

Shaman: The Mysterious Life and Impeccable
Death of Carlos Castaneda
by Mike Sager

Sarabeth and the Five Spirits: A Novel about Channeling,
Consciousness, Healing and Murder
by Beth Gineris

Meeting Mozart: A Novel Drawn from the Secret
Diaries of Lorenzo Da Ponte
by Howard Jay Smith

Death Came Swiftly: A Novel About the
Tay Bridge Disaster of 1879
by Bill Abrams

The Deadliest Man Alive: Count Dante, The Mob
and the War for American Martial Arts
by Benji Feldheim

Lifeboat No. 8: Surviving the Titanic
by Elizabeth Kaye

The Pope of Pot: And Other True Stories of Marijuana
and Related High Jinks
by Mike Sager

See our entire library at TheSagerGroup.net

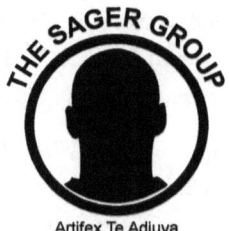

www.ingramcontent.com/pod-product-compliance
Lightning Source LLC
Chambersburg PA
CBHW031508120626
46545CB00005B/1790